TIME
of her
LIFE

MYRA HUNTER is a clinical psychologist who specialises in women's health. She has counselled women for many years and in the 80s carried out a major study to find out about women's experiences of the menopause. Currently, she is coordinating a large research project on women's health and well-being in midlife at Guy's Hospital Medical School in London, and is also working in the Department of Obstetrics and Gynaecology at University College Hospital, London.

Myra's first book, *Your Menopause*, was published in 1990 by Pandora Press and she is currently working on another, *Counselling in Obstetrics and Gynaecology*, to be published later in 1993. She is married with twin daughters and lives in London.

JEAN COOPE is a GP from Cheshire with a large family and a liking for music. She began research on the menopause in the 70s because her patients were interested in HRT, and has since published many original papers and pioneered an NHS clinic which offers screening and education to all middle-aged women in the practice. She is official spokeswoman on menopause and HRT to the Royal College of General Practitioners and a founder member of the Council of the British Menopause Society. Jean is married to Dr John Coope, a general practitioner who specialises in preventive health; her previous book, *The Menopause: Coping with the Change* was published by Optima.

Dr Myra Hunter & Dr Jean Coope

TIME
of her
LIFE

Menopause, Health and Well being

BBC BOOKS

To all the women who have been through our
clinics, helped in our research and whose voices can
be heard in the pages of this book.

ACKNOWLEDGEMENTS

The authors would like to thank all the women who have talked so honestly and
openly about their lives and experiences at their menopauses. A special thanks
to Suzanne Webber for commissioning the book and to Isabel Moore for making
the project such an enjoyable experience to work on. Myra Hunter would also
like to thank Lesley Bulman, Karen Liao, Jill Walker and Jim Jump for
stimulating discussions about midlife, and Sheila Lawler for typing the manuscript so
quickly. Jean Coope would also like to thank Joyce Marsh for her invaluable help
on her manuscript.

This book is published to accompany the BBC Education television series of the
same name which was first broadcast in April 1993

Published by BBC Books,
a division of BBC Enterprises Limited,
Woodlands, 80 Wood Lane London W12 0TT

First published 1993

© Dr Myra Hunter and Dr Jean Coope 1993

ISBN 0 563 36759 8

Editor: Isabel Moore
Design: Peter Butler
Illustrations: Nancy Sutcliffe
Charts: Mike Gilks and Peter Butler
Recipes created and tested by Lesley Waters

Photographs: Ron Sutherland p24; Tony Stone Worldwide/Dale Durfee pp38, 45,
Tony Stone Worldwide/Jon Gray p58, Tony Stone Worldwide/Don Bosler p85, Tony
Stone Worldwide/Ken Fisher p103; Sally & Richard Greenhill pp35, 51;
Format/Brenda Prince p57; Science Photo Library/St Bartholomew's Hospital p108;
Jean Coope p136; Photofusion/Janis Austin p169.

Set in Garamond No.3 and Gill Sans Light by Servis Filmsetting Ltd, Manchester
Printed and bound in Great Britain by Clays Limited, St Ives, plc
Cover printed by Clays Limited, St Ives, plc

CONTENTS

INTRODUCTION

This book is about changes and choices in midlife. The menopause is often seen as *the* change, but our middle years can witness changes in many areas of life: our career might take a new turn, so too might our relationships with family and friends, our role in the home, our leisure activities and self-image. Many of these can be changes for the better, but to make your own choices and positive adjustments you need information and facts – as well as time to think about them and the confidence to use them.

The menopause is one of the few remaining taboos that women face. Fortunately attitudes are changing. Women now approaching the menopause are part of a generation that has been much more frank about discussing their bodies – especially when it comes to fertility and child-bearing – along with their role at home and in society. These same women now want to know what to expect from the menopause, how to deal with symptoms, how to prevent health problems and what help is available.

Between now and the mid-1990s over 7 million women will go through the menopause in Britain. As part of the war and immediate postwar baby-boom generation, they will form a large and potentially influential section of the population. If you are part of this generation, male or female, or if you are in your 20s or 30s and are looking ahead, this book will provide you with the facts and practical advice that you need.

This book is also for those of you who are experiencing or have recently experienced the menopause and who may be adjusting to new roles at home and in the outside world. Post-menopausal women have their own particular concerns about health and ageing. We will give you the information and encouragement to help you to develop a full and rewarding lifestyle.

By describing the different experiences of many women we hope that you will find some to share, as well as some new perspectives and possibilities for your own life and choices.

Myra Hunter.

Jean Coope

CHAPTER ONE

CHANGES AND CHOICES

MIDLIFE IS BEING REDEFINED, PUSHED BACK AND EXTENDED. TEN YEARS AGO MOST BOOKS ABOUT MIDDLE AGE FOCUSED ON MEN AND WOMEN OF ABOUT 35 TO 55; IN THIS BOOK, WHICH IS AIMED PRIMARILY AT WOMEN IN MIDLIFE, WE ARE LOOKING MAINLY AT THOSE BETWEEN 45 AND 60.

Until fairly recently, menopause not only marked the end of a woman's younger, reproductive, years, it also heralded the start of her older years, the shortest and last part of her life. Things are different now. Women on average can expect to live until they are about 78 (that is, about 30 years after the menopause) and people in general are also staying younger for longer in terms of their attitudes and lifestyles. With improvements in diet, health care and living standards, the years between youth and old age can be very active and fulfilling. Not only is this a longer life stage but in the next two decades – because of the declining birth rate in the last 30 years – a greater proportion of the population than ever before will be of middle age and beyond.

Middle age suggests an emotional stock-taking, a reassessment of past achievements and disappointments, a time to adjust to new roles, for example with parents and children. It can be a time for reflection and also a time to make plans for the future.

Both sexes go through a process in middle age of weighing up life's gains and losses. For men it is a stage usually associated with the so-called male menopause, which seems to arrive around the age of 40. For women the picture is more complicated, for this same process of emotional stock-taking tends to be confused in people's minds with the menopause. The menopause is a biological event, but it is often blamed for a whole host of problems that are more to do with emotional and social upheavals. This is clearly unhelpful. So the aim of this book is to help you separate and clarify the influences and issues involved in the changes that might occur during your midlife.

Not so long ago we could assume that when a woman was 50 her children would be 20 and leaving home and that her parents would be 75 and nearing the end of their normal lifespan. Nowadays, however, these traditional stages are not followed in any fixed order. Some women still choose to marry young and have children early; others start a family in their late 30s and 40s. Today a woman's lifestyle is determined much more by her activities and aspirations than by her age. Of course ageing takes place. But this is a very gradual process, even though you might *notice* signs or *feel* older at certain times much more than others.

❝ When I was in my teens and 20s I thought that by the time I was 35 I'd be past it, wearing a twin-set and pearls, be working in an office, with two children. I have to laugh now I'm 46, in leggings and T-shirts, starting a course in computing with one child, a husband and a very active social life.

I never think of myself as middle-aged. It has such dull and dreary connotations – sometimes I don't even feel grown up! Seriously, I felt and looked older when I was in my early 30s, when my three children were young. I didn't have time for myself then. Now I take care of my appearance and have more money to spend on clothes. I think I'm much fitter and healthier these days.

It's strange isn't it. We divorced two years ago and since then my life has turned right around. It was possibly easier for me because we didn't have any children. It was hard, very hard at times, but I've learnt such a lot – small things maybe. I'm working full-time and I've made one or two close friends. They are very special. I sometimes feel lonely, but at this stage in life I feel what have I got to lose.

At my age (50) the advantage is that you have the confidence to be yourself, to look how you want to look – you spend all those years keeping a family going and in a way you have to lose yourself in a family, but now you can emerge and start a new life.

I've got a two-year-old and a six-year-old and I'm 45. I do feel rather older than some of the mums in the playground, but I think it's your attitude that's important. Sometimes I envy my friends who had children in their 20s – some are even at college now and are more or less off their hands. But the benefit to me of later pregnancies is that I established my career first. ❞

Get a group of 50-year-olds together and some may be grandparents, some may be dealing with adolescents, others starting exciting new relationships or embarking on a new career. Many do feel stressed, running a home and bringing up children and working, while some feel understimulated. On the other hand, a lot of women say they feel more confident at this age because of their greater experience.

This is a time when you can attempt to exert some direction and control over your life. Change nearly always brings

10

mixed feelings. For example, a sense of loss is often accompanied by fresh opportunities. So when children leave home, the initial sadness will often fade away once you begin to realise the extra freedom this will give you.

MENOPAUSE MYTHS AND EXPECTATIONS

Women are beginning to talk about the menopause more and more. But, like any taboo subject, it is still shrouded in myths, confusions and anxieties, leaving many of us uncertain about what to expect. In most Western societies the menopause passes without ritual or public acknowledgement. Information is gleaned from friends, relatives and media images of menopausal women, which often reinforce negative beliefs and unnecessary fears. Stereotypes and myths of menopausal women include the following:

△ the aggressive, garrulous older woman (the witch)

△ the forgetful, over-emotional, irrational and confused older woman (ruled by her hormones)

△ the depressed middle-aged woman with no useful role (on the scrap heap)

△ the embarrassingly over-sexed woman or one who has completely lost her libido (sex-mad or frigid)

△ the woman with hormonal or ovarian deficiency (she is ill).

None of these images is helpful to us in understanding the menopause. They typify the prejudice often felt towards older women in a society that overvalues youth, attractiveness and fertility, and fears growing old. Older women are expected to be caring, generous and motherly, so it can be a great shock when mum or gran reclaims her life and starts to think about herself for a change after years of putting other people first.

What is needed is a new image of a self-assertive 50- or 60-year-old woman, one who can take care of her own needs without running the risk of being labelled irritable, bossy or aggressive (see page 42 for more about assertiveness and how to be assertive).

11

So what <u>can</u> you expect to experience at the menopause?

△ The menopause is not an illness, but you can experience hot flushes and irregular periods. Some doctors, because they tend to see women with problems rather than those without, give the impression that the menopause is akin to a disease.

△ Your sexual feelings might increase, decrease or stay the same (see page 29).

△ Some women feel depressed during the menopause – but most don't. Recent research shows that depression is more likely to be associated with what is going on in your life than by the menopause or your hormones. (See page 37 for how to deal with depression.)

△ The menopause also gets the blame for many symptoms that have nothing to do with it. Headaches, aches and pains, depression, dizziness, tiredness and forgetfulness are often put down to the menopause, when stress and poor physical health are more common causes.

Many women – about one in five – have no symptoms at all during the menopause, while a similar proportion have problems such as hot flushes or vaginal dryness. This leaves the majority of women who go through some mild to moderate changes without too much trouble.

Studies of different cultures have found in general that the more older women are valued in a society, the less the emotional and physical impact of the menopause. In some communities, women even look forward to it: Mayan women in Mexico do, for instance, because it frees them from social taboos associated with menstruation and from years of continuous child-bearing. These women don't even have a word for hot flushes!

Cultural differences in diet, exercise and family size are likely to be important factors too. In Japan, women appear to be more concerned about age changes than the menopause itself, and they report far fewer hot flushes than North American and European women do.

All this suggests that our expectations and beliefs about the menopause are influenced by its social meaning for us and the

12

context in which we experience it – whether it heralds positive change or devalued status.

Here are the thoughts of a group of 45-year-old women in Britain talking about the menopause.

❝ *I wouldn't like to think I was going through the menopause, to be honest. I've got lots of friends who think they are and keep talking about all the awful things that can happen. It's not something I'm looking forward to, so I'm keeping it out of my mind till it happens.*

Well, I think I am menopausal. I don't feel particularly bad about that, but I am quite defensive about the pressures I believe are put on women at this time. I do feel strongly and quite angry about what I see as pressure to take HRT (hormone replacement therapy), for instance, and I feel annoyed that people seem to devalue older women and place a lot of emphasis on women looking young and decorative. The sort of built-in assumption is that once you start the menopause, you're not attractive and you have nothing left.

The thing that worries me is weight gain, a few extra pounds settling in the wrong places. I agree that it's wrong that women feel that they're not attractive after a certain age, but that's just the

society we're in. I think that it could make you feel worse if you felt that you could look better and you weren't making the effort. Weight gain would worry me.

I think it makes a difference to be informed – there are lots of aspects, physical and mental, that get confused. A lot of women don't ask, they just accept things or get the wrong information.

I don't think I've reached that stage (the menopause). I haven't got strong feelings really. It doesn't trouble me. I hope it just turns up and comes and goes quickly.

I'm very concerned about osteoporosis because my mother had it quite badly. (See pages 89 to 90 for facts about osteoporosis.)

Well, I don't know anything about it. I'm totally ignorant about it really.

In the summer I got pregnant and I've just had a miscarriage. Now I'm think-ing, how much time have I got left? I've got to wait for three months before I have another go, will I have time? There's a certain urgency, never having been preg-nant before. I've got no idea about the menopause at all. I don't feel I've got any signs, so it's all a bit of a muddle for me.

13

A lot of my friends talk about symptoms – irritability and hot flushes. I just wonder whether they're putting down to the menopause what's more to do with the fear of growing old. Some of them are having problems in their relationships, it's as if they're breaking up now, before it's too late! I don't know if the irritability is to do with their relationships or the menopause.

I'd quite welcome the menopause rather than have a period every three weeks. I have pains and heavy bleeding. I don't think the menopause is something where you think – that's it, I'm finished. It's just another stage isn't it?

I don't know if I'm starting it or not. Is it me being over-emotional? I've got grown children, 17 and 23, and my dad died four months ago. You've got a whole lot of problems at this age, haven't you?

Well, I've been diagnosed as having multiple sclerosis, so for me this is much more important. If and when the menopause comes I should sail through it – I sailed through the monthlies etc. If I need to go on HRT I'll go on it, if not I'll just try to keep as healthy as I can.

I don't see it as a problem. I think I'm in the menopause. My last period was three months ago. I do get hot flushes.

I'm not embarrassed by them, they don't really bother or overwhelm me. I just think it's something a woman has to go through. But I feel as though I don't completely understand what's happening. 🙶🙶

It's quite normal for women approaching the menopause to be unsure about what's in store for them. Younger women tend to have more negative ideas about the menopause than those who have been through it. Most older women are pleased to be free from menstrual periods and the risk of pregnancy.

The fear, held by some women, of numerous physical and emotional problems occurring during the menopause can, in fact, be self-fulfilling. Those who are particularly pessimistic tend, not surprisingly, to feel worse about their own menopause when it actually happens.

For many women the main concern about the menopause is uncertainty about when it will start, what will happen and how long it will last.

🙶🙶 *I see it as a transition. It's hard to know exactly what will happen in my case, but I'll be pleased when it's all over.* 🙶🙶

14

What *is* certain is that women of all ages need more information, not only about the menopause but about their health in later life. In a recent study of pre-menopausal women, over 80 per-cent wanted more information about it beforehand. We aim in this book to provide unbiased information to help you to form a realistic picture of what might happen, and to help you to be able to deal with changes that might occur. If you are well informed, you will also be able to weigh up the pros and cons of medical treatment in your case.

MENOPAUSE ISSUES AND EXPERIENCES

How you experience your meno-pause is very individual and might depend on many things, including:

△ your health and fitness

△ your sense of well-being

△ your hormone levels

△ your lifestyle (diet, exercise, stress)

△ your feelings about fertility

△ your age at menopause

△ your beliefs about it

△ the attitudes of those close to you

△ your level of knowledge.

Talk to ten different women who have been through the meno-pause, and you will get ten different points of view, not only about what happened, but also about how they viewed the changes and how they dealt with them.

❝ *I had several tries at IVF (in vitro fertilisation) but they didn't work. It took a long time and I was getting very stressed so we decided to leave it for a year so that my body could recover. My periods gradually stopped. I never thought it was the menopause – I'm 41 – so when the doctor told me I was just devastated. Now (eight months later) I'm still really in a state of grief.* ❞

Some women find it very difficult to deal with the feeling that their bodies appear to be out of control.

❝ *I am an orderly kind of person. My periods were always regular and my life is busy but, normally, manageable. Now that my periods are irregular and I'm getting these hot flushes and night sweats, I'm finding it quite hard. I don't trust my body. I'll be glad when it all settles down again. 99*

For others, the menopause represents a definite stage in life which marks the end of the reproductive years, or a time when the process of ageing looms large.

66 Thinking about my menopause, I did feel empty inside. For me motherhood, being able to have children, was very significant and I wanted to spend some time contemplating the years when the children were younger. I don't feel depressed but more thoughtful, as if I want to say goodbye to that stage before looking ahead.

What hit me was to do with ageing. Most people deny it but I think what women fear about the menopause is that it's a sign of getting older. No one real'y wants to get old. It's about facing death, and that needn't be a bad thing. It makes you appreciate life. 99

Women approaching or going through the menopause also ask many questions. These are often about their health in later life, as well as about HRT (hormone

replacement therapy), a treatment which has aroused much interest, even controversy, in recent years.

△ Do I need to use contraception?

△ Am I at risk of developing osteoporosis (thinning of the bones) in later life?

△ Should I have HRT?

△ I have a family history of heart disease, can HRT really help?

△ I feel depressed, is this the menopause?

△ Are there alternatives to HRT?

△ My periods are heavy. Is this normal?

△ I've gone off sex. Is this normal?

△ I don't want to use HRT. How can I cope with my hot flushes?

△ Does HRT improve your looks?

△ How should a 55-year-old woman look these days?

△ Should I tell my colleagues at work?

In the chapters that follow we will attempt to answer these questions and provide up-to-date information to help you to make your own choices and decisions. In some areas more long-term research is needed, but we will offer advice based on the current state of knowledge.

A TIME TO THINK

Time to think – about yourself – can be a rare gift in a woman's life. The menopause should be used, or redefined, as an opportunity for women to be contemplative, to look at their lifestyle, their health and happiness, and their relationships. The post-menopausal years can be fulfilling but are more likely to be rewarding if time and thought are invested during, or better still before, the menopause itself.

In the years preceding the menopause many women accumulate stresses at home and at work. Taking time to think requires delegating, saying no, and reversing some automatic responses.

Over the past century there have been huge advances in our understanding of the physical and medical aspects of the menopause. Energy has also gone into developing non-medical approaches and opportunities for women to discuss the menopause and midlife changes.

In many ways, the 1990s are a good time to go through the menopause. Women's health issues are now more openly and sympathetically discussed and, in general, women face less discrimination now than they did two decades ago – although there is obviously still room for improvement. We can expect that the menopause transition will become easier as a more self-confident and better informed generation of women prepares for it and passes through it.

CHAPTER TWO

LIFESTYLES AND LIFE CHANGES

CHANGES OCCUR AT ALL TIMES OF

LIFE, BUT FOR SOME WOMEN THIS IS

ESPECIALLY TRUE DURING THE TIME

WHEN THE MENOPAUSE OCCURS.

THINKING CAREFULLY ABOUT WHAT

IS HAPPENING WILL HELP YOU TO

MAKE THE MOST OF THE CHANGES

AND COPE WITH ANY DIFFICULTIES

THAT MIGHT ARISE — WHILE AT THE

SAME TIME RETAINING A STRONG

SENSE OF YOURSELF.

RELATIONSHIPS WITH YOUR PARENTS

Parents are growing older too, and we often face the loss of our mothers and fathers in our 40s and 50s.

66 My parents are in their late 70s and I'm 52. They are fairly healthy but obviously I know they can't live for ever. I see them more often now and we talk more than we used to. We remember things we did in the past. Having my own children makes me appreciate much more than I used to what they've done for me.

I've never got on with my mother. My father died two years ago – I really felt that. I feel ashamed that even at my age (55), I used to ring up and ask him what he thought about the news and big decisions I had to make, things like that. I miss him a lot. I visit my mother but there's always an edge. I think she resented my closeness with dad, felt left out by it. I still do my duty, of course, but I don't think we'll get any closer now. 99

Living with parents can be difficult, especially when there are differences in cultural expectations. Anna married Ramesh, who has an extended family in Britain, 30 years ago.

66 My husband's parents live with us. He is the eldest son and the family is very close, it's expected. I do find it hard. Ramesh (her husband) is very good but he is the go-between. It does put a strain on our marriage. My friends tell me not to do everything for them but they don't understand. I am beginning to compromise and insist on days off now and again. 99

Caring for unwell or elderly parents is often emotionally draining, quite apart from all the practical work involved. It can be hard to accept that these people who were once so strong are now dependent upon you. You may feel that there is no one left to look after you.

It can sometimes be helpful to talk with parents about the past. It might be the chance to clarify misunderstandings, to ask questions, and to express the things you have neglected to say. Some people feel the urge to make up a family tree – to fill in the details of relations while parents are still alive. However, some relationships have always been difficult and some conflicts may not be resolved before a parent dies. If you feel very distressed, bitter, resentful or angry with your mother or father it might be worth talking to someone (a friend or counsellor), to try to put the relationship into perspective.

" For years I was angry with mum. She seemed to favour my elder sister. She was more successful than me and did everything right; married, had children and now has given mum grandchildren. The thing is I adored mum more I think than Sandy (sister) did. It's strange really, last year I talked to mum about it. She said that she'd always tried really hard to treat us equally and that I was so envious of Sandy I'd spoil things on purpose. Looking back she did probably do her best – and seeing how hard my friends are finding it with children I can see it's not so easy. "

In childhood we tend to put parents on a pedestal, to see them as more powerful and more ideal than they are. Gradually they become not so perfect people in our eyes, especially when they become frail. It is important to respect their independence and individuality.

Many of us have in our early years taken in critical (as well as nurturing) parental messages, such as you don't deserve that, or you'll never succeed, you're too quiet, fat or thin, and so on. If such thoughts are still pushing you around in midlife this can be a good time to challenge them. Doing so can be quite liberating!

Remember, though, that you cannot look after others unless you take care of yourself. Harness the support of someone else (partner, friend, brother or sister) to help or even just listen, or to remind you to think about yourself as well. (See The Carers National Association, page 180).

When they are getting older parents may no longer provide a central pivot or meeting place for the larger family. For some women this can mean that they feel obliged to take over this role, while for others it might result in a feeling of separateness from brothers and sisters.

" My parents are both in sheltered accommodation. I visit when I can and so does my brother with his family. It's not the same though as it used to be. We used to have big family gatherings. I suppose I feel it more because I haven't a family of my own. "

Many women experience bereavement for the first time in midlife. Grief is normal and adaptive but requires time and energy – taking months or years depending

20

upon the relationship. There is often a natural tendency to avoid painful feelings by keeping busy, but don't overdo this. If you have had a previous loss, for example a relative in childhood, or a miscarriage or stillbirth, a bereavement can unexpectedly bring back those old sadnesses.

You may feel at times after a bereavement that your thoughts and feelings are so strong that you are losing your grip. Feeling like this can be part of grief (see the box below). Reduce some of the pressures and demands on yourself. Eat well, take as much rest as you can and exercise.

GRIEF: COMMON STAGES AND FEELINGS

▲ NUMBNESS AND DENIAL

not being able to take in fully that the person has died. Feeling confused; decision making should be delayed.

▲ GRIEF OR DESPAIR

now the painful strong feelings come to the fore; depression, anger, blame, regret or guilt. These often come in waves. You may feel empty inside, tired and have difficulty sleeping. It is common to think the person is still alive and to have vivid dreams. It is as if your whole body is having to readjust and under-stand what has happened. You may not want to see many people for a while. Knowing that this is part of a process which affects each of us differently can help you through this stage.

▲ RECOVERY OR LOOKING AHEAD

gradually the loss is accepted. It may still be painful to think about the person and reminders may provoke feelings but they become more manageable and less over-whelming. You adjust to life without the person and it becomes possible to look to the future.

21

Having people around who listen and understand is valuable, and if you have no one do not be embarrassed about seeking help. There are now many facilities for bereavement counselling (see the listings at the end of this book).

Being in touch with the extremes of life and death can help us to put other problems into perspective and to appreciate what we have and make the most of the future.

RELATIONSHIPS WITH YOUR CHILDREN

Contrary to popular belief, children leaving home – the empty nest syndrome – is as often tinged with relief as with sadness for parents.

The two boys are 19 and 23 now. Tony and I rarely have time to ourselves. It's a constant battle to get them to help. Sometimes it feels as if I'm running some kind of hotel. Sean (the older one) is trying to get his own place but, you know, it's hard for them to make a start. He really should have left home by now.

When Tom and Katy left home – they're both married now – I kept their rooms as they were. I had to stop myself going round to see them all the time. The house was so quiet. But last year we changed the house around and we made a combined study and exercise room and a spare room out of the children's rooms. Now I wouldn't have them back!

In fact, women whose children have left home tend to be more satisfied with life and less likely to be depressed than those actively engaged in childrearing. The physical and emotional demands of young children are never-ending, especially if you are a single parent or don't get much help at home from your partner. The stresses of balancing the needs of home and work and organising childcare, as well as other activities, can be exhausting. Many women find the responsibilities and the social pressures to be superwoman too much.

I was taking Sophie and Jack to school and playgroup, swimming once a week, to gym and football, doing housework each day and working part-time in a solicitor's office. I had to be there – there was no leeway. I shared a nanny two mornings a week. Honestly, I just got more and more stressed, spending most of my time in the car trying to meet time deadlines; I thought it was partly because

I'm an older mum. In the end we sat down and looked at the whole picture and made some useful changes. Really, what was I trying to prove? A gym class was not worth the aggravation to my mental and physical state! 99

Enabling children to become independent can be as much of a challenge as the responsibility of caring for them, especially with adolescents who are often awkward to deal with.

66 *Now I've learnt to stand back a bit, let them make their own mistakes – as long as they keep to our rules when they are at home. There's not an awful lot I can do about what they get up to when they're away but they know what our views are.*

I thought that there would be less of a generation gap between me and my kids than there was between me and my parents. In a way it is better – there have been fewer changes. But I do think as well that the children themselves need to see us as older and old-fashioned. 99

Dealing with teenagers is inevitably fraught at times. Having a strong parental unit, or friends to compare notes with, can help. Strength is needed to stand firm and to enable the child to de-velop and separate. As children grow up, mothers in particular can find that they have to make adjustments. You may have to shift from a pattern of putting others' needs first (often essential with very young children) to giving priority to your own.

Avoid taking up positions of martyrdom – such as being a dogsbody to your teenage children and their friends who pop in and out at all hours of the day and night. This is likely to result in resentment later on. It is helpful and reassuring for children to see that your tolerance has limits and that you have other interests and commitments.

Grandparenthood can offer the fun and intimacy of contact with young children without the hard work. This can be particularly welcome if a grandchild is born when you are aware that you can no longer have children yourself.

66 *My daughter's children are a joy to me – a breath of fresh air. I feel a sense of achievement as well. More so, I think, because my son has mental health problems and it's hard not to blame myself for that.* 99

It is also quite common to feel uncomfortable at times. For

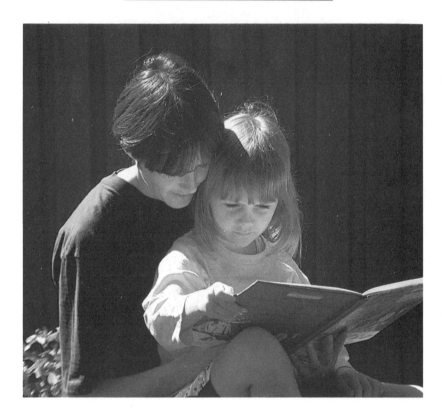

Having your children late can definitely help to keep you young. Enjoy your time together – you'll find that you will learn as much from them as they will learn from you.

example, feeling jealous of time spent with the other grandparents, wishing your daughter or daughter-in-law would do things differently, or wanting to be more or less included. Acknow-ledge these feelings. Be open with your children – ask them how they want you to be and tell them what you would like. Avoid blaming and complaining. It is a time for adult negotiation and mutual respect. Similarly, if you have done enough baby-sitting this week, say so and don't feel guilty!

For those without children the end of the child-bearing years can be a mixed blessing.

24

I'm 41 now and have had several tries at infertility treatment. I think we have given up hope really. I do feel sad about it but in a strange way the menopause would be a sort of relief – the whole issue would be over. People would stop asking me whether or not I'm going to have children.

I've never really wanted to marry. I have close friends of both sexes. I thought at one time I might have children but I'm not that bothered. But when you ask me about the menopause – yes, I think I might feel some regret. Not about not having a specific child but the choice is taken away isn't it.

RELATIONSHIP WITH YOUR PARTNER

We have been together now for 26 years. When we were bringing up the boys (now 19 and 22) and both working, life just seemed to carry on – with ups and downs – on its own momentum. Recently we've had to start to look at what our interests are, how we spend our time together and, perhaps more important, in what ways we are different and have needs that the other can't satisfy. We are much closer now.

We are brought up on this ideal of romantic love and it causes a lot of problems.

My first husband and I divorced six years ago. I met Joe last year. I have learnt from the mistakes in my marriage and with Joe I feel that the relationship is more equal. I don't want to remarry though – we have our separate places and I feel I need that independence and personal security.

Individuals inevitably change over the years. For people in long-term relationships these changes exert pressures which require thought and adjustments, but for some it is only later in midlife that difficulties surface. On the other hand, there is often now the time to give your relationship more attention.

A common problem is for conflicts to arise when one partner undergoes changes in attitudes.

I had tended in the past to be quite dependent on Martin, but gradually over the years, and with my success at work, I have more confidence now, more faith in my own judgements. I want to go out more and he wants a quieter life. It does cause a bit of tension. I think we've got a lot of compromises to make.

It can be frustrating when you're trying to present a new image to the outside world only to find that your partner fails to acknowledge that you are any different. Change can lead to insecurity and can be seen as rejection, so it is important to talk, explain and re-assure about anxieties that are unwarranted.

It is often said that during midlife there is a crossover in interests and aspirations: women become more assertive and outward looking, while their partners, who may have been the main wage-earners for most of the relationship, become more inward looking and home-centred. There may be some truth in this especially as more women now seek fulfillment at work and in their own social lives.

This will not be the case for everyone, however. Divorce and remarriage are increasingly common and more people are remaining single than before. There may be more lifestyle options today, but these very personal choices such as divorce or separation are never easy to make, and some people are constrained by financial dependence.

All relationships are unique, but the following are common problems or themes voiced by many women in their 40s and 50s.

DISILLUSIONMENT – There is the realisation that your partner is not ideal. Romance has waned. You love each other but wonder if this is enough. This feeling can be compounded if you are feeling older and less attractive. For some, love may need to be rede-fined. Hollywood images of idea-lised relationships have a lot to answer for. A degree of disap-pointment may be a natural reac-tion which requires a mature appraisal of the situation. The important thing is not to lose sight of what you do have.

“We have had a terrible time lately. It's as if we're both asserting our rights at home and competing over space and time. You think you've got things sorted out and then something else comes up. But I do value the warmth between us, the sense of having the shared past and someone knowing you so well. It's just as though you need to take a fresh look from time to time.”

BOREDOM AND LACK OF INTIMACY – Habits and over-familiarity can make for an easy, tolerant rela-tionship. But it is not surprising that engaging in mundane house-hold tasks day after day, year after year, can detract from inti-macy. Paradoxically, for closeness to develop you need to see each other as separate people again. Make an effort to make the time that you do spend together enjoyable. Having new or separate interests helps, as can reorganising household chores and responsibilities.

RESENTMENT AND CONFLICTS – Some relationships seem to be built around quarrels. These may be expressed in terms of who does what around the house, about a past affair, about money or sex. If they are frequent or are worsening, you may well question whether you want to continue in the relationship or whether it can be improved. Often the arguments reflect insecurities in both parties which are difficult to talk about. There may be misunderstandings arising from the way feelings are or aren't expressed. And some people find that they repeatedly form patterns in relationships which are unhelpful.

Reappraisal in these situations is not easy. Start by looking at yourself. Are you blaming your partner for behaviour that you are at least partly responsible for? Set time aside to talk, and have a basic rule to be constructive. For example, 'I would really like it if

you suggested social activities' sounds much better than 'You never (or why don't you ever) suggest anything'. The latter is too general and accusing.

Remember that everyone is vulnerable in a way, and fears of rejection and humiliation are more or less universal. It is unrealistic to expect to have all your needs satisfied by another human being. Many people seek help and find that counselling can improve communication, whether you intend to stay in the relationship or not. (For Relate, see listing at the end of this book, and for talking about the menopause with partners see page 52.)

The United Kingdom has one of the highest marriage rates and also one of the highest divorce rates in the European Community. Fewer divorces occur in the over 45 age group however; it is couples between 16 and 34 who have been married for five to nine years who are the most likely candidates for divorce. Interestingly, widowers and divorced men are much more likely to remarry than divorced women. For some women then it could be a case of once bitten twice shy!

Nevertheless, separation and divorce are significant life events which may result in feelings akin to grief, especially if a separation happens suddenly and the decision is not mutual. Anger and blame are common reactions. You may feel depressed, which is understandable in the circumstances.

It is helpful, if you can, to maintain a balance between anger and total blame of the other person on the one hand, and self-blame and depression, on the other. Use anger to mobilise your life. Reflect on your contribution to what went wrong and try to avoid repeating mistakes in future relationships. Many women also feel a sense of relief when an unsatisfying relationship ends, especially if they have experienced arguments and bad atmospheres at home with little physical or emotional contact for several years.

❝ It took me quite some time to get my confidence back. You feel rejected in all aspects of yourself. Talking to my sister and friends helped a lot. I make an effort to think about my good qualities. I've lost weight and bought new clothes. People say I look better. I still have fond feelings for him. But it would never have worked. I don't think we'll ever be close friends but I can see him now without

getting upset. I do have definite plans for the future – the sense of freedom is much stronger than I'd expected!

My main worry was the children – they're all in their late teens. We hadn't got on for years really. I'd kept things going for the the children. It's funny. They knew more than I'd thought. When I finally decided I'd had enough and told them, they said they understood and that we'd be better off living apart. They'll still see John (her husband). It was such a relief to know they felt OK about it. ❞

Separation happens without choice for women whose partners die. The painful feelings ease with time (see page 21) but this is cold comfort when surrounded by a profound sense of loss and daily reminders of it. Having contact with friends, family and support groups does help. For bereavement counselling agencies see listing at the end of this book.

Of course many women remain happily single, being involved in relationships at times, while retaining their independence. Today many more people in Britain are living alone than was the case 30 years ago – and the trend is increasing.

❝ I know I couldn't live with anyone now. I have friends and I have a relationship with a man now but I enjoy my own space too much. ❞

RELATIONSHIPS WITH FRIENDS

❝ Quite an important part of my finding myself has been spending time with other women. Talking, seeing how they deal with problems has helped, as well as going out together. I go running every week with a friend. It's relaxing mentally and physically. ❞

Friends can provide a different perspective, encouragement, the opportunity to share experiences, as well as companionship. The latter is important as it can often be difficult for women to go out alone.

❝ I have four friends, one is divorced, two are bereaved and one never married. We met at an evening class – all learning French. Now we see each other at least twice a week and we're all going on holiday together later on this year. ❞

Frequently outliving their partners, many women in their 60s and 70s gain support and enjoy fulfilling relationships with each other.

❝ I meet Iris and Anne every week at a tea dance and we arrange to go out for dinner every month or so. We know that we can rely on each other. We are different in many ways but being in our late 60s there is a lot to share – about the past as well as the present and future – I hope!

The sort of friendships I have made in the last ten years or so with women are different from the rather stormy relationships I had with my two husbands. They are much more easy going and accepting and we have a lot of fun. ❞

SEXUALITY

In many ways a sexual relationship can be more enjoyable as you get older – women are considered to be at their sexual peak in their 30s and 40s. If you have experienced your menopause, contraception is no longer needed (see Chapter Five), and this can encourage you to develop the self-confidence to be more sexually demonstrative as you get older.

As with other aspects of life, studies of women's sexual behaviour during midlife reveal a range of experiences. Some clearly have active sex lives, and this is particularly the case for those who have always enjoyed their sexual relationships and those who have

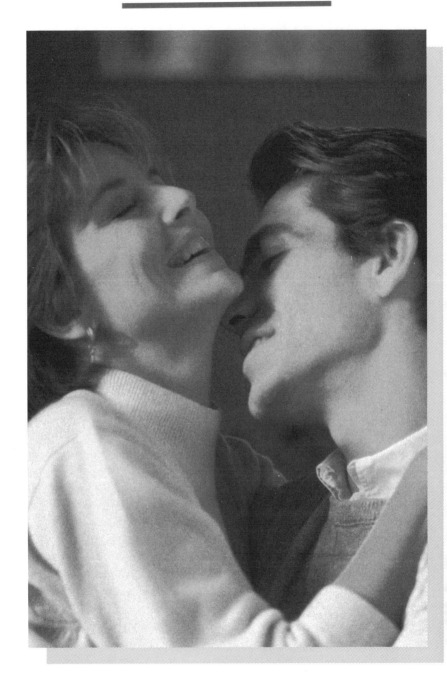

begun new ones. Most sexual relationships get better or stay the same, but for about one in three couples sex becomes less satisfying or less important.

In general, and for both sexes, sexual interest tends to decrease gradually with age. This may reflect biological changes as well as the relative importance of sex compared with other components of a relationship in later life. Physical problems, such as joint stiffness or weakness after a stroke, can interfere with sexual enjoyment; for practical advice see page 33. Excessive alcohol intake can also disrupt sexual functioning, especially for men.

If you are less interested in sex than you want to be, the following reasons may be worth considering.

HABIT AND FAMILIARITY – In long-term relationships it is easy to take sex for granted, to slump into bed exhausted, expecting your partner to make all the effort. Privacy may have been invaded by the proximity of

Flirting with your partner can be fun at any age! Don't be afraid to show affection – and he won't either.

children, and stresses and tiredness sap available energies.

FEELING UNATTRACTIVE – If your role is limited, to childcare for example, you may have less opportunity to see yourself as a sexual being, reflected back through the eyes of others. Seeking more adult company can help, as can paying more attention to your looks and body. If you're feeling negative about yourself follow the ideas suggested in the box overleaf.

SEXUAL INHIBITION – Once patterns have been established in sexual relationships it can be difficult to alter them. Despite the greater frankness about sex, we are still exposed to confusing images of our sexuality. Many men still hold conflicting ideas about women – as Madonna and whore. Then there is the tendency to see your own (female) sexuality through men's (or the media's) eyes. All this has inhibited women's natural ability to discover their own desires. Attitudes may be changing, but there are still negative stereotypes of the older sexual woman. There is no alternative to asking or

NURTURE YOURSELF

▲ Treat yourself to body lotions, relaxing baths, massage

▲ Swim or exercise regularly to increase awareness of your body

▲ Eat healthily and well

▲ Notice your thoughts about your body. If you are telling yourself I'm too fat, ugly or the wrong shape – make efforts to keep your body healthy but don't be too self-critical; challenge these views too.

showing your partner what you (do or don't) want. You don't have to be young to be sensual – in fact the reverse is often the case!

CHANGES ASSOCIATED WITH THE MENOPAUSE – The menopause does not have a major effect on women's sexuality, but if you find it difficult to come to terms with emotionally, or if you expect to lose sexual interest, then any anxieties might well dampen your sexual feelings. Your partner's attitude will also play a part.

Some women experience vaginal dryness at the menopause which can make penetration uncomfortable, but there are ways of alleviating this problem (see page 87). Night sweats (hot flushes at night) can make physical proximity less appealing! Most couples can deal with this kind of problem reasonably easily if they understand its cause.

In fact, despite these changes, the majority of sexually active couples continue to be satisfied with their sexual relationships during the menopause.

PARTNER'S SEXUAL INTEREST – A woman's menopause is often blamed for a flagging sex life, when her partner's interest or sexual functioning is just as important. The male menopause does not exist as a biological event, but men can have greater difficulty in maintaining an erection with age, especially if they are stressed or experiencing mixed

32

feelings about their own age and achievements.

66 It's ironic isn't it. Now that I'm enjoying sex more – taking longer over foreplay and feeling more relaxed, John (her partner) is finding that he can't wait that long. It's as if our timing is all wrong. We have to laugh about it. 99

With openness and sensitivity these changes can be adjusted to. But if you find that anxiety and expectations of failure are interfering, you can try some simple suggestions used in psychosexual counselling (see below). Or if your problems feel too entrenched going to a counsellor may help (see listings at the end of this book).

Other causes of lack of sexual interest include depression, anxiety and ill-health, so it's worth checking to make sure that these are not to blame. Stress and marital problems are the commonest however.

And of course it goes without saying that if you and your partner are happy without an active sex life then that's obviously fine too.

REDUCING SEXUAL ANXIETY AND INCREASING COMMUNICATION

▲ Learn to relax

▲ Don't necessarily aim for penetration or intercourse

▲ Take time to relax together and spend time touching and stroking each other – aim to enjoy receiving and giving in turn. Don't aim to be aroused or for your partner to achieve an erection

▲ Gradually include genital areas, communicating through touch what pleases you.

These stages can help to diffuse anxiety about performance; many sexual problems respond to this graded approach.

WORK

❝ My work is my saviour. It's the one place where I feel valued. I am a personnel administrator — I've worked my way up and know the ropes. There's a good atmosphere in the office and I can get things done.

My job is insecure. It's a worry — they're making people redundant and who knows whether I'll be next. It would be very hard for me to get another job at my age (56). I resent it too; at home (India) I was brought up to expect not to have to work by now and to live as part of the family. Here it's not like that, my husband and I divorced 10 years ago and I have to work to support myself these days.

When it's going well it's fine. But when there's too much pressure at work or problems with one or two of the managers, I start to feel tense. I know I shouldn't take responsibility for their problems but I want to make everyone feel OK like I do at home.

I worked for 15 years as a secretary — full-time and part-time. Then in the last year I started a drama course. At first everyone thought I was mad. But it's done me the world of good and you never know — I might be able to put it to use one day.

I think it's hard for older women — they are not given the same respect and promotion as men are at the same age. Things are getting a bit better but you know men still like to feel they have the power over young women around them. ❞

On average two-thirds of 45- to 60-year-old women in Britain work full-time or part-time. Work can bring challenge, reward or stress and conflicts at any age. But in midlife some women feel that opportunities are more limited or that their skills and abilities are not sufficiently valued, while others have reached the peak of their careers or are pursuing new directions.

There are now more role models of successful women, but some feel that expectations of women are too great.

❝ Women of our generation have such high standards — to have a career, be lively and interesting, be a good mother, and in the end working at home too. I've got friends who have opted out of all this and deliberately taken less demanding jobs. It's a compromise. ❞

It's important to find a job that can give you a sense of satisfaction — but won't leave you too stressed to cope with the rest of your life.

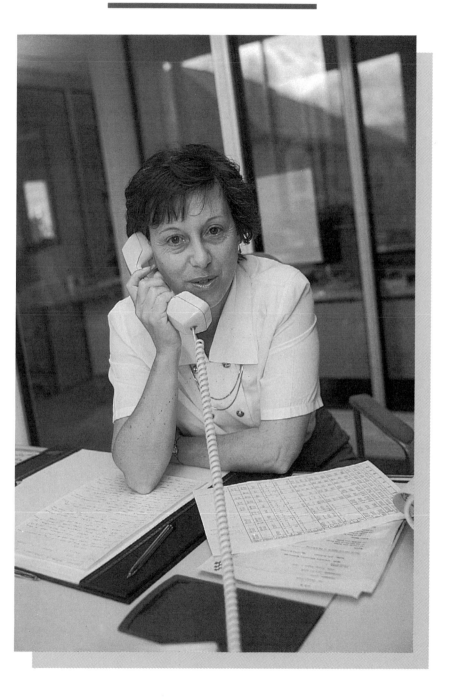

Women who work have, on average, much less free time than working men. Some families adjust well to a woman's career by sharing or reversing roles to a degree.

❝ I'm a doctor and earn a lot more than my husband. It's quite practical really, his job is less demanding so he does more of the shopping. It was a bit of a shift at the beginning but it makes sense doesn't it? He thinks he's a new man but I'm not so sure about that! ❞

Unemployment is a source of stress for women and men. Financial hardship brings obvious practical problems and having to seek work repeatedly can get you down. However, for a lot of people, midlife is a time when financial pressures are relieved.

❝ We are much better off now that most of the mortgage is paid off, and the boys have set up homes of their own. I remember when I had to watch every penny. Now I can enjoy shopping and we have more choice of holidays and hobbies. ❞

Retirement can be more flexible these days and many women retire earlier while others choose to work beyond retirement age.

❝ It's wonderful, the best years of my life. I'm busy. My only regret is that I didn't have much time before my husband retired. We have learnt to give each other space but at first we got on each other's nerves a bit.

The best thing I've done since I turned 60 has been to learn to drive. It might be harder at my age but it's worth it. ❞

There are now many more leisure facilities available for people of all ages – as well as opportunities for travel, learning and retraining.

❝ Lots of women I know have learnt skills that they are using at home, for example, word processing, designing, teaching music. It's as if the distinction between work and hobbies becomes less at this age. I'm lucky, I've got a good pension so I do have that security.

I worked for years in the same office. It was well paid and I supervised the other staff. But the monotony got to me. I paid for a careers guidance interview. They looked at my range of skills in different areas of my life. That was very good for my confidence. I'm considering retraining now. ❞

For information about retraining, returning to work and education courses see pages 179 and 180.

BUT HOW DO YOU FEEL?
Emotional and physical symptoms, particularly depression, are
common signs that lifestyles are
too stressful or that there are
problems which should be tack-
led. Recent surveys have found
that single women tend to be less
likely to be depressed, while
younger women who are married
with young children suffer more.
Women are more likely than men
to experience depression by a
ratio of two to one. This is
especially the case for women
during the reproductive phase of
their life.

There is no strong evidence to
support the idea of 'menopausal
depression' – low oestrogen levels
alone do not cause depression.
Women are not more likely to be
depressed after the menopause. In
fact many are much happier!

Studies following large
numbers of women through the
menopause have found that the
main causes of depression for
middle-aged women when it does
occur are:

△ life stresses – at work, marital
and family problems, caring for
elderly parents, and particularly
bereavements

△ social problems – financial
insecurity

△ ill-health – affecting oneself or
family member

△ having very pessimistic views
about the menopause or the
future

△ long-standing emotional
problems.

Obviously, everyone feels low at
times, but if you have the following symptoms or feelings a lot of
the time:

△ wake early and sleep badly for
the rest of the night

△ poor appetite

△ lack energy and interest in things
you used to enjoy

△ feel profoundly sad that life is not
worth living

△ feel guilty and blame yourself,

and if you feel unable to deal
with them yourself, you should
probably get help from your
doctor or seek counselling (see
page 178).

Is it the menopause?

If you are going through the menopause and feeling low or irritable, these feelings may be a normal reaction if you are having severe hot flushes or night sweats that disturb sleep (see page 86 for how to cope). Some women say that they feel more emotional when hormone levels are fluctuating, but this is usually the case only when there is a *rapid change* in hormone levels, for example, after a hysterectomy with removal of the ovaries, which does seem to lead to tension and depression for some women.

❝ *I had my ovaries removed when I had my hysterectomy. I felt drained afterwards – really low, tired and drawn. I don't know if it was the operation but I certainly felt different after I had it, until I started hormone treatment.* ❞

It is also easy to notice and label feelings – that occur for other reasons – as being to do with the menopause. It can be easier to blame the menopause, for example, for feelings arising from difficult problems like an unhappy marriage. Or you may not be depressed but contemplative.

❝ *Stan says that I've been moodier lately. But I think that there's a gap between how others see you and what is really going on. I mean I think I have been more reflective in the past two to three months, to try to understand it (the menopause). It may mean that I haven't been quite as keen to do what everyone else wants to do so I may have come over as being bad tempered, but that isn't how I feel. I don't feel depressed either – I've done quite a lot of thinking and I just need time.* ❞

Facts and feelings about the menopause are discussed in greater detail in Chapters Three and Four, and for how to deal with problems that may arise, see Chapters Four and Five. But remember that most women do not become distressed when their periods stop – so don't *expect* to feel bad.

ARE YOU STRESSED?

Recognising that you're under stress is an important step. It is nothing to be ashamed of. We all have our stress threshold. Headaches, excessive tiredness, lack of concentration, angry outbursts, panicky feelings, tension and tearfulness are common signs.

Stress is difficult to describe. It is not entirely internal

COPING WITH STRESS

When faced with a difficult situation do you tend to:

HELPFUL REACTIONS

▲ Let feelings out, talk to friends.

▲ Go over and over it until you understand the situation.

▲ Go back and try to deal with the problem.

▲ Take active steps to avoid the situation recurring.

▲ Let people know how you feel.

LESS-HELPFUL REACTIONS

▲ Avoid thinking about it.

▲ Blame everyone else.

▲ Worry constantly.

▲ Hold feelings in.

▲ Withdraw from family/ friends.

▲ Eat more/less.

▲ Use drugs, alcohol.

TEMPORARY SOLUTIONS

▲ Treat yourself to something, for instance, go out for a meal

▲ Bottle it up then break down

▲ Keep busy

▲ Distract yourself

▲ Cry on your own

or external but an interaction of the two. One helpful definition is: When you feel that the demands of a situation (or lifestyle) cannot be met by your abilities or resources. What is stressful to one person may not be stressful to another. And apparently positive changes, such as holidays or moving house, can be stressful too.

It is often the accumulation of demands that creates a feeling that you can't cope. Something happens, like having building work done in your kitchen, that becomes the last straw in an already busy lifestyle. Women tend to invest emotional energy in maintaining and dealing with family relationships and their work often goes unseen. As a result it's not uncommon for them to underestimate the demands in their day to day life or feel that they shouldn't complain. If you are busy working the effects of over-stress may only be noticed at times of enforced rest.

66 It was when I went into hospital for the operation (removal of fibroids) that I realised how things had been getting me down. I'd cry for the least thing and had dreams about everything collapsing around me. 99

This woman's sister had recently died of breast cancer. She had not felt able to take time off to grieve for her.

Coping with stress

If you do feel stressed, answering these questions might help you to pinpoint some of the causes so that you can begin to make some changes:

Q *First, do you give yourself time to think about your lifestyle?*

A If the answer is no, start by giving yourself permission to take some time for yourself (even if it is only half an hour in the evening) with no other demands on your time.

Q *What is most stressful for you?*

A It could be a particular event (a parent is ill), conflicting demands from people around you (husband and children), accumulation of worries, a difficult relationship or a combination of factors. Elicit the help of someone else – a friend or counsellor – who might offer a different perspective.

Q *Is your view of the situation you are facing accurate?*

A For example, faced with learning a new task at work such as computerisation of your office, would you tend to think, 'I'll never manage, it'll mean extra work, I won't have the time', or 'I know it might be difficult at the beginning but I learnt to type and if others can do it so can I'. The latter will make you feel better and is probably fairly accurate.

Q *How do you normally cope with stress?*

A Examples of helpful and less helpful ways of dealing with stress are shown on page 39. If stress is acute then temporary solutions can bring relief, but chronic stress usually requires more active coping strategies.

Q *How can you try to solve the problem?*

A It can be helpful to brain-storm all possible solutions regardless of how crazy they may seem; other people may see options that you have overlooked. If you have identified possible solutions, make them specific and attainable. For example, one woman found that coming back to her home in the evening after work and being faced with two hungry adolescents set the wrong tone for her for the rest of the evening, so she decided to give them definite tasks like laying the table and preparing some food. These were exchanged for pocket money so that she could sit down and relax with a cup of tea for half an hour when she came in.

Some goals may be long-term, such as changing jobs, but it is helpful to build in short-term goals too.

Q *Do you have ways of relaxing?*

A If you haven't, remember there are now many facilities to help people to relax. Yoga classes, active sports or evening classes can be equally relaxing. You may just enjoy sitting undisturbed in front of the TV for an hour. It is a matter of finding something that is right for you. Some relaxation exercises are described on page 165.

" *I am very busy but I found going to the cinema once a week relaxing. A good film distracts me and I sleep well afterwards.*

The best thing for me is a hot relaxing bath. **"**

Making changes usually involves letting other people know what you want and don't want, and sometimes what you would like them to do for you.

BEING ASSERTIVE

Being unassertive is a complaint voiced about many women, as is dealing effectively with angry feelings. Often anger is bottled up or inwardly directed, leading

ARE YOU UNASSERTIVE?

▲ Do you say sorry more often than you need to?
▲ Do you have difficulty in saying no if someone asks you an unreasonable favour?
▲ Do you tend to put yourself down to make others feel comfortable?
▲ If you feel angry do you say nothing and take it out on someone else?
▲ Can you express affection and receive compliments?
▲ Can you let someone know that you disapprove of something without being overwhelmed by anger?
▲ Do you harbour resentment over long periods of time?

If most of your answers to the above questions are YES, practise and rehearse being more assertive in some of the above situations. Be aware of:

▲ eye contact – don't avoid looking at people
▲ posture – sit or stand firmly – don't cower!
▲ tone of voice – speak loudly enough
▲ facial expression – if you are saying something serious, then look serious
▲ emotions – try to keep calm
▲ communication – give a simple, unambiguous, clear message, and repeat firmly if necessary.

to self-blame, low self-esteem and tension. Assertive people communicate self-respect. They are able to receive and give compliments and say what they want firmly and politely. So be prepared to say, 'We seem to disagree here', or if being pressed to make a difficult decision, 'I'll think about it and let you know as soon as I can', rather than being badgered or confused into doing or agreeing something you don't want to.

SELF-IMAGE

Feeling good and looking good usually go hand in hand. If you value yourself this shows, and not only in your outward appearance – it is also reflected in your mood, your health and your whole image. But we often have conflicting attitudes towards appearances and this is particularly true in midlife when we are presented with only extreme stereotypes of older women.

Clothes, make-up and hairstyles are all modelled for us on much younger women. And by showing these to us in this way we are encouraged to believe that ageing should be feared. So do we grow old gracefully or fight the ageing process?

❝ I want to look attractive, who doesn't. But if you are seen to be spending a lot of time on making the most of yourself you're in danger of being seen as vain, insecure or cheating.

I do make more effort now, with make-up and exercise, to look better. I don't see anything wrong with that. You see 40-year-olds who look dowdy and have let themselves go. It's such a shame. It's partly to do with age but it's much more to do with caring for and about yourself.

People nowadays seem to hold their age much better. Looking at photographs of my mother at my age, she looks much older than I do.

Most of my friends have been brought up to have values that would go along with the idea that we should age naturally and not be ashamed of a few wrinkles. It's difficult though: they would use a henna hair rinse but wouldn't consider dyeing their hair or having a face lift. ❞

You don't need to aim to reclaim youth in order to look good. But it can be helpful to take some time to think about your image in your 40s and 50s. Who am I? How do I want to look? Will I still be me after the menopause?

43

Most of us have an internal sense of self that goes back to childhood and adolescence. You will have added layers of experience and developed certain qualities while under-using others. Taking a fresh look at your ideas about yourself can therefore be revealing; maybe your self-image could do with an update. For example, one woman looks back.

❝ *I always saw myself as shy. Once you have that view it's difficult to shake it off. Now I'm functioning very well at work and with friends. It's time to throw away that label.*

I love music but was never very good at school. Now I've got more time – and I'm aware that if I don't do it now I never will – so I've taken up piano lessons. People get too fixed in their minds; you can do most things if you try. ❞

Try saying: I am a woman who has the following qualities

....
....
....
....
and unused potentials ....
....
....
....
Fill in the spaces for yourself.

Similarly many of us stick with the same make-up or choices of colours and clothes without taking time to reassess.

❝ *I wear much brighter colours now than when I was younger and take more time getting the right accessories.*

I went to a large store and had a make-up session. The woman there was very helpful and told me to use paler foundation colours for my skin, to go for pinky brown eyeshadow instead of blue and to avoid blusher. We tried different lipstick shades. I'm very pleased with the result. I rinse my hair regularly. I use a lighter colour, though, than my original hair shade. It looks much better on me.

I really don't feel that I have to conform to an older woman's look. Things are changing. My friends are in their 40s and 50s and wear jeans as well as smart suits. ❞

Some changes that women describe – such as middle-age spread – need not be inevitable if you take up exercise and eat healthily. Smoking is bad for

You don't need expensive haircuts and lots of make up to look good – feeling good about yourself can do the trick too.

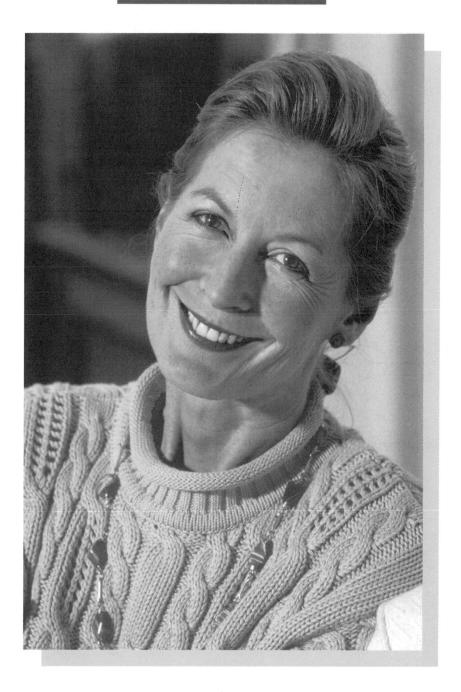

both health and skin, so this is a good time to stop or at the very least cut down dramatically.

The menopause can threaten that sense of continuity of a woman's self-image. If you are having hot flushes and irregular periods your body can feel very different, but these changes are temporary. Part of taking time to think means redefining yourself as a woman who no longer has periods and cannot have children. And making positive choices about how you want to be in the future.

If you think of your reproductive years (from about 18 to 48) as the first half of your adult life you have the second half (48 to about 78) to look forward to. It is worth giving yourself some of the attention that you have probably directed to others until now. Looking after your inner self – your health and well-being – is as important as caring for your outer appearance. Here are some tips for both.

INNER SELF

△ Eat a healthy diet (see page 62)

△ Take regular, enjoyable exercise (see page 55)

△ Drink lots of water

△ Stop smoking

△ Learn to relax (see page 165)

△ Try to reduce stress

△ Believe in yourself

△ Take risks and make new plans

OUTER SELF

△ Have a good haircut (older women today have more varied and flattering hairstyles than ever before)

△ Keep fit

△ Protect skin from sun's rays and use a moisturiser to keep the skin supple (skin creams cannot take away wrinkles but moisturisers applied to still moist skin plumps them out and protects the skin)

△ Facial exercises may help to tone up sagging chins and cheek muscles

△ Skin tone can become paler with age so make-up may need to be lightened to adjust too.

Skin does become thinner with age and wrinkles are often the first signs of ageing. Brown marks and age spots gradually become more common. There is some evidence to suggest that HRT (hormone replacement therapy – see Chapter Six) might help to firm the skin by increasing the amount of collagen in it, but HRT will not get rid of wrinkles. (Collagen forms a bed of tightly packed fibres supporting the skin and it helps to maintain the skin's elasticity.)

Vigorous exercise also stimulates blood flow to the skin, which in turn keeps the skin's collagen fibres well-nourished. Collagen needs regular circulation to keep fresh. So skin massage as well as regular physical exercise should help.

A final ingredient is vitality. Attractiveness is obviously more than looks. Being interested in other people, pursuing ideas, reading and taking up new activities can generate fulfilment, and may ultimately be more rewarding than admiring glances!

CHAPTER THREE

PREPARING FOR THE MENOPAUSE

PREPARING FOR THE MENOPAUSE MEANS BEING INFORMED, CHALLENGING THE MYTHS AND TALKING ABOUT WHAT ACTUALLY HAPPENS. IT ALSO MEANS TAKING STEPS TO IMPROVE YOUR HEALTH AND WELL-BEING SO THAT THE SECOND HALF OF YOUR ADULT LIFE IS EVEN BETTER THAN THE FIRST.

WHY PREPARE?

The menopause has been veiled by misinformation, embarrassment, shame and fear. It reminds us of ageing – another taboo. This is probably why it's hard to talk about, and why, as a result, fears persist unreassured. Fears about losing looks and sex appeal and becoming irrelevant are common. Men on the whole know very little about the menopause and women often deny its impending arrival.

Information gleaned from mothers and from media stereotypes may add to existing fears. But if your mother had a bad time it does not mean that you will. And the medical profession hasn't helped either: by focusing on HRT (hormone replacement therapy), they may have created the impression that a woman who does not take HRT is destined to have a whole host of physical and emotional problems. This is an overly negative picture which is unhelpful to those who do not need, or choose not to have, HRT.

Another fear is that the menopause strikes at a single point in time – that you will suddenly change drastically and unpredictably overnight. This is, for nearly every woman, *not* the case – a natural menopause is a gradual process of adaptation.

These myths and fears are the very barriers to the knowledge that can banish them. Most women today would readily agree that it makes sense to prepare for childbirth, an experience which most look forward to. The benefits of information, breathing exercises and emotional and physical preparation include having less anxiety, better health and greater control over the event. It is surely time that we applied these principles to the menopause.

If you approach the menopause not knowing what to expect, the physical changes may be misinterpreted.

❝ *When I first began to have hot flushes I'd no idea what they were. I had palpitations and I really thought there was something wrong with me. I used to have bouts of anxiety after I had the children and I thought my agoraphobia was coming back. I can't tell you the relief I felt when the doctor told me that it was the menopause.*

All I knew about was hot flushes. My periods stopped quite suddenly really and I thought – great, I'm over it! Then a few months later during lovemaking I didn't respond like I used to. I felt as keen as before but there was less moisture. It wasn't the sort of thing I'd go to the doctor with. In the end, after a few months of feeling bad, I talked to a friend who gave me a book to read. It all fitted into place then – I'm using a lubricant and it's fine now. ”

In a recent study of women living in south-east England, those who believed that the menopause brought numerous physical and emotional problems were more likely to feel depressed when they reached their own menopause. This distress can be avoided if you are approaching yours, and you prepare for it.

CHALLENGING THE MYTHS

The first step is to take some time to look at your own beliefs. Imagine a menopausal woman in your mind's eye. How does she look? What is she like? How do you feel about her? Then visualise yourself as going through the menopause – this can be difficult, so take your time.

Repeat the exercise with a friend. Check your thoughts and feelings against the common myths. Be honest with yourself and acknowledge your fears. Where did they come from? Your expectations may have been influenced by friends or members of your family, or you may just have absorbed our general

MYTHS AND STEREOTYPES

ABOUT THE MENOPAUSE

- I will lose my looks
- I will get depressed
- I will go mad
- I will age overnight
- I will be less feminine
- I will lose my sex appeal

ABOUT AGEING

- I will have no energy
- I will put on weight
- I will become introverted
- I will be lonely
- I will be less active
- I will be unsociable

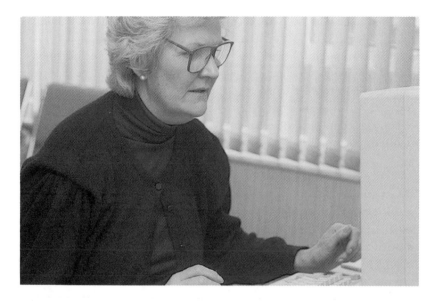

cultural attitudes towards older women.

Very few people want to age. But many of us tend to have overly negative ideas and stereotypes about being older. Older women need *not* be inactive, introverted, overweight or lonely. If you are in good health, there is no reason why you can't have an active and fulfilling life well into your 70s, 80s or even 90s. It is probably necessary to face your fears and personal images of your menopause and to challenge these before you go on to envisage a more realistic and positive self.

Visualise yourself again five or ten years from now – how you

Another myth to ignore: it's just as easy to come to grips with modern technology when you're older!

might look, your self-confidence, your interests and activities.

Be aware of other people's reactions when you start to talk about the menopause. You may well meet jokes, embarrassment and comments like, 'It's nothing to do with me', when you start to talk with friends and family. Don't give up! If you overcome these barriers most people are keen to know as much as possible.

Because the menopause is so individual, you will find people drawing on the experiences of one or two women who have had terrible problems, or who may have just sailed through it. You should put these particular stories and experiences into a broader context. Be brave and start talking about the menopause from an informed perspective.

BE INFORMED

Information can help you to have realistic expectations and to know what the changes mean, as well as what you can do if problems arise. This involves understanding the physical changes that occur (see Chapter Four), and which problems might be to do with the menopause (hot flushes, vaginal dryness) and which are more likely to be caused by other factors like ill-health, stress or ageing (wrinkles, headaches, depression).

Get to know your own and your family's medical histories. Become familiar with your lifestyle habits – which may result in health risks, as well as benefits (see Chapter Five). Pinpoint those that you might be able to change, such as smoking, diet, overwork, from those that you cannot such as height or skin tone. And think about the medical and non-medical treatments that are available if you should experience problems.

Clearly, it's impossible to be totally prepared. As many women know from the experience of childbirth, the unexpected can happen. Nevertheless, it's reassuring to know that there is help available for most problems. And it is important that you don't blame yourself if you approach the menopause fit and healthy and then experience severe hot flushes. An open-minded attitude is probably most helpful.

❝ *I prefer not to take pills and I have a good diet and go to keep fit once a week. I wanted a fairly natural childbirth – this happened with my second child but not with my first – with him it was epidural, forceps, the lot. So I suppose now I'm thinking that for the menopause, again I'll do what I can for myself and see what happens. If it's bad and I can't cope then I might well have HRT. I'll wait and see.* ❞

EDUCATE YOUR PARTNER

The onus is on you to educate your partner. He will not understand unless he is informed about the menopause, about your feelings and about the changes that you may want to make.

Mentioning the menopause to men brings mixed initial reactions.

❝ *I talked to my husband about it. I don't know if he was trying to be nice to me. He said that his main concern would be the health side, whether I kept well. He wondered if I'd get depressed because I'd had post-natal depression, and I said that there was no reason why I should. He felt that it would be good for him to know and be prepared.*

I've just started the menopause I think. My periods are irregular. I'm in a relationship at the moment and he's younger than me. It's a bit difficult to talk about it. I tried to bring it up and he says, well, you're in the menopause – what's the big deal? He doesn't see me as any different really.

My husband reacted really strongly. He practically walked out of the room. I think he wants to see me as still young, you know. I think he's going through a male menopause, and thinking about me as menopausal makes him feel older.

He was vaguely interested but I didn't want to make it into a big problem. We've had other medical problems. I've told him about it. I think if nothing dramatic happens there'll be no great reaction. ❞

Most men know very little about the menopause. Some may see it as a reminder of their own ageing. Many of them will be going through adjustments of their own. If this is the case with your partner, it can be a chance to open up a discussion of his feelings too. Talking together about the menopause may make it easier for both of you to deal with any changes that do arise.

❝ *I'm 52 and have had hot flushes for two and a half years. Malcolm does know about them, by trial and error really. He knows to give me a seat by the window and tries not to get annoyed if the duvet is on the floor in the morning.*

I think I have changed with the menopause. Not in a physical way but in my attitude to life. Now I've got more time to myself and a bit more money, I feel much more independent. It's that that he's having to get used to! ❞

It seems likely that the generation of men now in their 40s, many of whom have been interested and involved in childbirth, will in turn be keener than past generations to understand the menopause. But your partner won't if you don't tell him how you are feeling about it.

53

LIFESTYLE CHANGES

The relative health risks for women after the menopause are not usually known or discussed. For example, heart disease is the main cause of death in women after the age of 50, and fractures resulting from osteoporosis interfere with the quality of many older women's lives (see Chapter Five).

Preparation for the menopause means attempting to reduce your chances of developing these diseases, as well as preparing for a healthy and happy second stage of

LOOK AT YOUR LIFESTYLE

TRY TO

▲ STOP SMOKING — and be generally healthier and look better; smoking is a risk factor for most health problems. It's also very ageing.

▲ TAKE REGULAR EXERCISE — and feel in shape with more energy; exercise reduces your risks of heart disease and osteoporosis and improves your sense of well-being.

▲ EAT WELL — and, in order to reduce your risk of heart disease and osteoporosis, eat healthily; if you need to lose weight and you do, you'll feel better.

▲ REDUCE STRESS — and feel less depressed and anxious; reducing stress means that you'll be less affected by hot flushes and have better relationships with others (see pages 164 to 166 for ways of relaxing).

▲ PAMPER YOURSELF — and give yourself treats, because altering habits can be difficult. Mark your change of life positively.

adulthood. This should not be self-punishing but rather part of a wider approach of looking after yourself and your emotional and physical needs.

There are many individually small things that you can do that, collectively, can have a significant effect on the quality of your life.

Stop Smoking!
There are many simple things you can do to break your smoking habit – for instance, here is our eight-point plan:

△ First make up your mind. Your decision is the most important part. Think of yourself as a nonsmoker.

△ Set a date. Plan the first day carefully.

△ Change your routine. Avoid situations in which you have a strong urge to smoke, or do something else such as deep breathing. Use nonsmoking areas when you go out.

△ Take one day at a time and be pleased with yourself. Enlist the support of family and friends.

△ Remember that the strong urge for a cigarette only lasts a short time and then *passes*. The urges will become less frequent with time.

△ Practise refusing cigarettes and saying I don't smoke – with pride!

△ Give yourself regular weekly or monthly rewards.

△ Keep active and learn to relax.

There are immediate benefits to your health if you give up smoking – you'll see and feel them almost at once. Even if you don't succeed in giving up entirely, try to persevere and at least cut down the numbers you smoke. Every little helps a bit!

Take Regular Exercise
Most people know that they should exercise more than they do. But another popular myth is that the need for exercise decreases as we get older.

NOTHING COULD BE FURTHER FROM THE TRUTH.

All our bodily systems need to be used to function well, and many of the aches, pains and stiffness commonly associated with age can be alleviated by exercise. Sedentary lifestyles, under-exercised muscles and under-used bones are much to blame for health and weight problems in midlife.

The main challenge is to find the right kind of exercise to fit easily into your lifestyle; the benefits far outweigh the extra effort you will make. For example, exercise can:

△ burn off some excess calories which will help you lose weight and feel better

△ improve your mood

△ improve your posture

△ increase energy and stamina

△ reduce aches and pains

△ help you to sleep better

△ improve your circulation

△ improve the efficiency of your heart and lungs

△ keep your bones healthy and so help protect you from osteoporosis

△ help to fight off stress.

Nearly everybody will benefit medically from even a small amount of exercise. It's never too late to start!

Different types of exercise are good for different things, although any type will have a beneficial overall effect on your health. Some useful ones are:

TO STRENGTHEN YOUR BONES – exercise needs to be weight-bearing, that is involve pull and stress on the long bones of your body. Skipping, aerobics, dancing and brisk walking are all weight-bearing. It's best if this type of exercise is practised during the time that bones are growing, so encourage your family and younger friends to do them with you.

It's not clear how much exercise is needed to maximise bone

Exercise isn't just about staying healthy and feeling better, although it's important for both; it's about doing things with a friend as here.

56

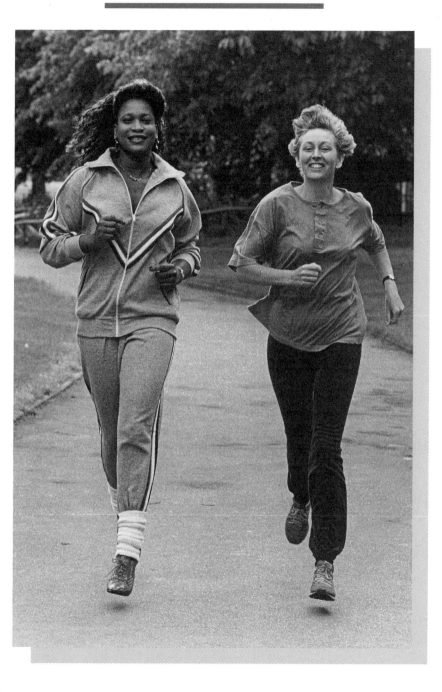

strength. Some experts say that 20 minutes three times a week is about right, although studies of post-menopausal women also suggest that those who have a generally active lifestyle are less prone to bone fractures.

Brisk walking and aerobics have similar protective effects and brisk walks might be easier to fit into a busy lifestyle. Swimming is not weight-bearing but increases suppleness and strength so you may choose one or two types of exercise that complement one another.

❝ I go swimming with a friend once a week. It's for social reasons as much as exercise. It's relaxing and I always feel better afterwards. I have brisk walks in the park twice a day – the dog makes me do that!

I'm not the type to join a class. But what I have found helpful is an exercise videotape. I put it on for half an hour in the evenings when my husband goes out.

Well I'm worried about my partner's health as well. So I persuaded him to

Tennis can help you meet people and feel better too.

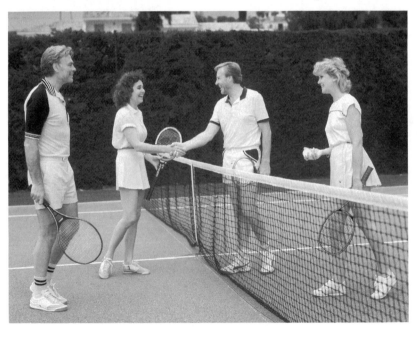

join a badminton club with me. I'm also getting him to come to a dance class as well. 🙦

FOR YOUR HEART AND LUNGS – aerobic exercise strengthens the muscles of your heart and lungs and increases stamina. This type of exercise should be vigorous enough to make you breathe more quickly and increase your heart rate, and the best activities are those that make you slightly out of breath and keep you moving for 20 minutes or more: running, brisk walking, cycling, aerobic classes, skipping, squash and swimming. (As you can see, some exercise is both aerobic *and* weight-bearing and is therefore particularly beneficial to do.)

When doing aerobic exercise, wear suitable shoes and maintain a good posture. Breathe deeply. Start off gradually and don't over-do it. Exercise should be built up slowly and if in doubt talk to your doctor about the kind of exercise for you to begin with. For instance, if you have a history of heart disease, jogging would not be suitable for you.

PELVIC FLOOR EXERCISES – (also called Kegel exercises) tone up your pelvic 'floor', the group of muscles which support the bladder, bowel and womb. Exercising your pelvic floor muscles also increases blood flow to your vagina and by doing so keeps it moist and healthy. Other benefits include reducing the likelihood of stress incontinence and vaginal prolapse; some women find that they also increase sexual pleasure.

If you have had children you may be familiar with these exercises. To identify the pelvic floor muscles – the *pubococcygeus* – imagine a figure of eight around your vagina and anus. To tighten them, push upwards as if you are holding in a tampon or stopping yourself from passing water. Hold the muscles tight for a few seconds then release them. Repeat several times. After a while you can draw up the muscles a little, stop and hold a bit longer – and then relax.

Once you have mastered the technique these exercises can be practised anywhere – several regular short bouts a day are recommended – for example, in the shower, at traffic lights, or whenever you have a cup of tea!

🙦 *I do my pelvic floor, leg and stomach exercises in the bath every evening.* 🙦

To FEEL GOOD – regular exercise can promote a feeling of well-being or give a mental tonic. It seems to be short and sustained bouts of vigorous activity, such as aerobic exercises, that are especially beneficial for mood. One explanation for this might be that exercise increases the output of chemicals called endorphins in the body which naturally produce a feeling of euphoria. Again, regular exercise is best. It also helps you to sleep and can provide a welcome distraction from daily concerns.

❝ *I go regularly to modern dance classes. It's amazing – there are women of all ages. I feel transported from my work pressure, housework and shopping for those precious 45 minutes or so. It's great.*

Swimming is best for me. When I was 55 I had a stroke affecting my right side. I felt embarrassed at first but now I'm much more confident and the exercise is really good for increasing my strength.

I love fell-walking – it's difficult living in a busy town, but every weekend and on holiday we go on treks. Even my son and his girlfriend are getting keen on it now. I think it's addictive!

My aim when I retire is to walk the coastal path as far as I can around Devon and Cornwall. I'm getting in training already. It's not just the exercise at all – it's the scenery. It's just something I've always wanted to do. ❞

One approach to exercising is to think of activities you enjoy and see which of these is compatible with exercise. It may be tap-dancing, taking an early evening walk, or walking to work twice a week. Set yourself realistic goals to begin with. And it is worth thinking through any obvious barriers that might interfere with your plans, such as having to travel too far to an exercise class, or depending on someone else for a lift.

It's important not to over-exercise since women who do, such as marathon runners, can suffer from amenorrhoea (loss of periods), which leads to lowered oestrogen levels and bone loss. However, few women have this problem!

After you exercise, always take time to relax.

If you have any kind of disability which might make the exercises described above difficult, contact The British Sports Association for

DON'T EXERCISE	STOP EXERCISING IF YOU
If you feel ill, have a cold or flu	Become uncomfortably breathless
In extreme heat or cold	Break into a cold sweat
For a couple of hours after a heavy meal	Feel dizzy or faint
If you've been drinking alcohol	Have chest or leg pains.

the Disabled (see page 179) for information and advice. EVERY-ONE can do some exercise!

Healthy Eating

Eating a healthy diet is a crucial part of caring for yourself at any age. And if you aren't already doing so, now is the time to start. It needn't be complicated but it can require some thought. Women often tend to make sure that their children eat well but then neglect their own dietary needs. Some simply have acquired bad habits.

❝ I go all day on cups of coffee and a roll at lunchtime. By the time I get home, sort out the dinner, it's half past seven. I'm starving then and I must admit I spend most of the evening picking at bits and pieces to relax. ❞

Look at what you eat and the way you eat and be honest with yourself. You may need to make some adjustments, perhaps to reduce the amount of fat or salt in your diet or to eat more fresh fruit and vegetables. Many people are eating more healthily than they used to. In the past 30 years some aspects of the British diet have changed dramatically, for instance consumption of eggs has halved and the intake of butter has fallen by three quarters. But the British diet, in general, still contains far too much animal fat. Healthy food *need* not be more expensive or time-consuming to prepare; pasta and wholemeal sandwiches are good substitutes for fried foods, for instance, and the fresh juice of an orange tastes better than a fizzy drink.

GUIDELINES FOR A HEALTHY DIET

Eat a varied diet made up of fresh, unprocessed and unrefined foods from the following groups:

▲ Fresh fruit and vegetables for vitamins, nutrients and fibre; eat raw when you can, or lightly steamed.

▲ Wholemeal breads, pasta, cereals and pulses (beans and lentils) for fibre, protein, vitamins and minerals.

▲ Milk, cheese and yoghurt for calcium for your bones.

▲ Fish, meat, poultry and eggs for protein; include oily fish, no more than one or two eggs a week and cut the fat off meat.

▲ Drink lots of water rather than soft drinks.

▲ If you are a strict vegan, make sure you get enough B12 vitamin.

▲ Use oils such as sunflower or olive for cooking and for salad dressings.

Calcium is essential for bone formation. Exercise increases bone strength but this only works if you have enough calcium in the first place – and you need it throughout life to build up bone. So educate your younger sisters and daughters!

Before menopause women need approximately 800 milligrams (mgs) of calcium per day, while for post-menopausal women the requirement increases to at least about 1000 mgs. Many women need to increase their calcium intake at this stage of their lives, therefore, and this can easily be done by making slight dietary changes. If you are unsure whether *you* need to do this, keep

Try to cut down on:

▲ Salt – which increases your blood pressure and water retention.

▲ Refined sugar in cakes, biscuits, sweets – these put on weight and contain no nutrients.

▲ Animal fats – which raise blood cholesterol (bad for your heart and arteries); steam instead of fry and use vegetable oils.

▲ Coffee – too much causes sleeplessness and tension.

▲ Alcohol – if you are drinking more than 14 units per week (one unit = a glass of wine, half a pint of beer or one measure of spirits).

A sample daily menu could be:
▲ **Breakfast** – orange juice, muesli and milk, tea.
▲ **Lunch** – beans on wholemeal toast, yoghurt, or a wholemeal sandwich.
▲ **Dinner** – wholemeal vegetable spaghetti or vegetarian lasagne with Parmesan cheese, mixed salad, fruit salad or strawberries.

a diary of what you eat for a week and roughly work out your calcium intake. Increase your intake if necessary and repeat.

Many women have cut down on dairy products because of their high fat content, but skimmed milk is now very popular and actually contains more calcium than full cream milk. If you are allergic to dairy products or if you are a strict vegan, use soya milk that has been fortified with calcium and vitamins. Most non-meat-eating vegetarians will probably get enough calcium in their diets, as long as they eat or drink some dairy products; nuts, dried fruit and leafy green vegetables are good sources of calcium too.

If you want to make sure you are getting enough calcium, you could take calcium supplement in the form of tablets – they're widely available from chemists and health food shops.

To be properly absorbed calcium needs vitamin D which is normally formed by sunlight and found in fish liver oils, fortified

CALCIUM RICH FOODS

(in mgs per 100g, about 3½ oz, of food)

Dairy	Calcium	Vegetable/Fruit	Calcium
Cow milk (¼ pint)	180	Parsley	330
Skimmed milk (¼ pint)	195	Spinach (boiled)	600
Natural yoghurt	180	Watercress	220
Cheddar cheese	800	Chick peas	140
Cottage cheese	60	Beans (haricot)	180
Edam cheese	740	Beans (kidney)	140
Parmesan cheese	1220	Dried figs	280
Cream	79	Broccoli	100
Egg	52	Tofu (bean curd)	507
		Lemon (whole)	110
Fish		**Nuts**	
Tinned salmon	195	Almonds	250
Tinned sardine	460	Brazil	180
Fried whitebait (eat small soft bones)	860	Muesli	200
		Sesame seeds	870
		Peanuts	60

Meat and white fish contain very small amounts.
Bread, flour and cakes also contain calcium (100-150 mgs per 100g.)

milk products and many multi-vitamin preparations. Most people will get this from their diet and outdoor activity, but if you are bedridden or have a very limited diet, you may need a supplement; do discuss it with your doctor if you feel you do.

Remember, though, that too much vitamin D is toxic and should be avoided. Women with any serious chronic illness or kidney disease should check with their doctors before taking any supplements.

Excessive amounts of alcohol and caffeine can interfere with bone metabolism, and smoking is particularly damaging to bone health. In general, we tolerate alcohol less well with age, so if you are feeling ill-effects it makes sense to cut down. If drinking is a problem see listings at the end of this book for organisations that can help.

Making the Changes

Making changes to your routine should not be overly punishing. Many women have a love-hate relationship with food. Very strict diets usually don't work – and some slimming diets can be dangerous. If you eat for comfort and feel bad afterwards, try to decide on a healthy diet and let yourself enjoy it. Enlist the support of a friend or partner. But if you need help to change or if you have a particular problem such as binge eating or anorexia, or if you are very overweight, do seek help. See listings at the end of this book for suitable counselling services and organisations.

Set yourself realistic and specific targets and monitor your progress daily or weekly. For example, aiming to cut out sugar in tea and coffee is much better than a general aim such as to eat fewer sweet things. Give yourself encouragement and rewards. And if you relapse, don't give up! For some, group activities such as exercise classes, health clubs or meetings arranged by organisations are excellent ways to make changes. Or you may prefer to meet with a couple of friends to encourage one another. There are several menopause self-help groups in Britain which offer information and group meetings – ask at your local health centre or library if there is one in your area; there is no reason at all why women approaching the menopause can't use them as well. If there isn't one, why don't you start up a group of your own.

CALCIUM-RICH RECIPES

It's often difficult to conjure up interesting meals when you're faced with a bald set of ingredients and their nutritional content, so to start you off where eating calcium-rich foods is concerned, we offer the selection of specially created recipes that appear over the following eight pages – all of them easy to cook and absolutely delicious to eat.

CHICKEN AND BROCCOLI CHOWDER WITH CHINESE SESAME NOODLES

This marvellously filling soup is a feast in itself.

Serves 4

CHOWDER

1 tablespoon olive oil
4 lean smoked bacon rashers, rinded and diced
2 cloves garlic, crushed
6 boneless chicken thighs, cut into strips
1 leek, finely sliced
6oz (175g) mushrooms, wiped and sliced
1 teaspoon chopped lemon grass or strip of pared lemon rind
1 bay leaf
8oz (225g) potatoes, peeled and grated
¼ pint (150mls) white wine
1½ pints (900mls) vegetable stock
Salt and freshly ground black pepper
4oz (100g) frozen sweetcorn
1lb (450g) broccoli, trimmed and broken into small florets
Chopped fresh parsley

SESAME NOODLES

2 teaspoons sesame oil
1 tablespoon olive oil
2oz (50g) sesame seeds
6oz (175g) thin egg noodles, cooked

First make the chowder. Heat the olive oil in a wok or a large saucepan, add the bacon and fry for 1 minute. Stir in the garlic and chicken strips and fry for a further 30 seconds. Add the leek, mushrooms, lemon grass or lemon rind, bay leaf, grated potatoes, wine and stock. Season well, bring to the boil and simmer the soup for 20–25 minutes, adding extra stock or water if necessary.

Add the sweetcorn and broccoli florets to the soup and simmer for a further 6–8 minutes, or until the broccoli is just tender. Season to taste.

To make the sesame noodles, heat the sesame and olive oils in a wok or frying pan, add the sesame seeds and fry until they are lightly toasted. Add the noodles and toss well over a fierce heat for 2 minutes. Season well.

To serve: Add the parsley to the chowder and ladle into large soup bowls. Heap a spoonful of noodles into the centre of each bowl and serve immediately.

TORINO BAKED PASTA

Cooking pasta, potatoes and kale together may sound odd, but don't be put off – this is both easy to prepare and absolutely delicious to eat! If you can't get kale, or you don't like it, any other greens, such as cabbage or spring greens, can be used instead. Serve with Watercress, Spinach and Carrot Salad (see page 69) for a satisfying and healthy meal.

Serves 4

1lb (450g) potatoes, cut into chunks
(keep the skins on)
8oz (225g) curly kale, chopped
8oz (225g) dried pasta (wholemeal
and green)
2 tablespoons olive oil
1lb (450g) tomatoes, skinned and
thickly sliced
2 cloves garlic, crushed
1oz (25g) butter
1oz (25g) flour
2 teaspoons grainy mustard
½ teaspoon ground nutmeg
¾ pint (450mls) milk
1 bunch of fresh thyme,
finely chopped
4oz (100g) grated Parmesan cheese
Salt and freshly ground black pepper
2oz (50g) cheddar cheese, grated
2 tablespoons dried breadcrumbs

Pre-heat the oven to gas mark 6 (200°C/400°F). Boil the potatoes until just tender, remove from the pan and then par-cook the curly kale in the water from the potatoes. Drain and refresh under cold water. Cook the pasta in boiling salted water until just cooked (al dente). Drain and refresh the pasta under cold water.

Heat the olive oil in a frying pan, add the tomatoes and garlic and cook over medium heat for 30 seconds. Put to one side.

Melt the butter in a small saucepan, add the flour, mustard and nutmeg and cook over gentle heat for 30 seconds. Remove from the heat and pour in all the milk, whisking until the sauce is smooth. Return to the heat, stirring continuously until the sauce thickens. Simmer for 4–5 minutes and season to taste. Stir in the thyme leaves.

Put the pasta, potatoes, kale, tomatoes and Parmesan cheese into a large shallow ovenproof dish, stirring well to mix, and season with plenty of freshly ground pepper. Spoon over the white sauce then scatter over the cheddar cheese and breadcrumbs. Bake in the oven for 35–40 minutes or until the dish is crisp and golden on top and bubbling hot.

Serve immediately.

ORIENTAL SPICED FISHCAKES WITH CUCUMBER RAITA

Make these as spicy as you like, and serve with noodles. Tinned salmon or sardines are ideal for this recipe.

Serves 4

FISHCAKES

1 × 14oz (400g) tin red salmon
1 tablespoon olive oil
1 onion, peeled and chopped
1 tablespoon desiccated coconut
½ teaspoon ground nutmeg
1 teaspoon ground coriander
A few drops of Tabasco sauce (or to taste)
1lb (450g) boiled potatoes, mashed
1 egg, beaten
Dried brown breadcrumbs
Olive oil for drizzling
1 bunch of watercress (to garnish)
1 orange, cut into wedges (to garnish)

SAUCE

1 tablespoon olive oil
1 clove garlic
1 bunch of spring onions, trimmed and chopped
1-inch piece root ginger, peeled and grated
2oz (50g) black-eyed beans, cooked
2oz (50g) chick peas, cooked
1 × 14oz (400g) tin chopped tomatoes
4 tablespoons soy sauce
1 teaspoon brown sugar
½ pint (300mls) water

CUCUMBER RAITA

½ cucumber, grated (with the skin on)
½ pint (300mls) natural yoghurt

Pre-heat the oven to gas mark 5 (190°C/375°F).

First make the fishcakes. Drain the liquid from the tinned salmon and mash the flesh in a bowl. Heat the olive oil in a frying pan, add the onion and fry gently until softened. Stir in the coconut, nutmeg and coriander and cook for a few minutes more. Tip the contents of the pan into the salmon, adding the Tabasco sauce, mashed potatoes and the beaten egg. Mix well until all the ingredients are combined.

Sprinkle your work surface with dried breadcrumbs and divide the salmon mixture into eight roughly equal portions. Using the breadcrumbs, form each portion into a round, arrange on a plate and chill well in the refrigerator for 30 minutes. Remove from the refrigerator and arrange the cakes on an oiled baking sheet, then drizzle a little olive oil over each one. Bake in the oven for 25–30 minutes or until they are crisp.

While the fishcakes are cooking, make the sauce. Heat the oil in a saucepan, add the garlic and half the spring onions and cook for 1 minute. Stir in the ginger, beans, chick peas, tomatoes, soy sauce, brown sugar and water. Season well, cover and simmer for 20–25 minutes.

To make the cucumber raita, mix the cucumber and yoghurt together and set aside.

To serve: Remove the fishcakes from the oven, arrange them on a large

68

plate and garnish with watercress and orange wedges. Add the remaining spring onions to the sauce, check the seasoning and serve it separately in an attractive jug or bowl. Serve both with the raita.

CABBAGE AND WALNUT (OR HAZELNUT) RAGOUT

This is a delicious way to cook an everyday vegetable. Serve with warm crusty bread, either your own (see the Tomato and Sage Bread recipe on page 72) or bought. If you can't find red cabbage, green or white or spring greens can be used instead.

Serves 4

1oz (25g) butter
1 tablespoon olive oil
1 small red cabbage, trimmed and shredded
1 onion, peeled and sliced
2 pears, quartered, cored then sliced
1 clove garlic, crushed
$\frac{1}{4}$ pint (150mls) beer
6oz (175g) toasted walnuts or hazelnuts
6oz (175g) Roquefort cheese, crumbled
4oz (100g) mature cheddar cheese, grated
Salt and freshly ground black pepper

Melt the butter in a wok or frying pan, then add the olive oil, cabbage, onion, pears and garlic. Toss over high heat for 2 minutes, add the beer, cover the pan and cook over medium heat until the cabbage begins to wilt and soften (this will take about 4–5 minutes). Stir in the chopped nuts and cheese, tossing briefly to allow the cheese to melt and coat the cabbage.

Season to taste and serve at once.

WATERCRESS, SPINACH AND CARROT SALAD

This superb salad takes only minutes to prepare and makes an excellent snack lunch served with home-made bread (see our Tomato and Sage Bread recipe on page 72); or serve as an accompaniment to pasta dishes.

Serves 4

SALAD
1 bunch of watercress
4oz (100g) fresh spinach leaves
3 large carrots, peeled and grated
DRESSING
1 tablespoon poppy seeds
The juice of 1 orange
1 tablespoon natural yoghurt
4 tablespoons olive oil
Salt and freshly ground black pepper

To make the salad, gently combine the watercress, spinach and grated carrots in a salad bowl. Mix all the dressing ingredients together then season to taste.

Trickle the dressing over the salad just before serving.

GRAPEFRUIT, ONION AND TOMATO SALAD

This unusual combination of ingredients makes a refreshing snack, salad lunch or delightfully different accompaniment to strong roasted poultry, such as duck or turkey.

Serves 4

2 pink grapefruit
3 beef tomatoes
1 large onion, peeled and finely sliced
Salt and freshly ground black pepper
$\frac{1}{4}$ pint (150mls) olive oil

Using a sharp knife, cut away the peel and pith from the grapefruit. Slice them across into rounds and place in a bowl with any juice. Slice the tomatoes into thin rounds, then arrange the grapefruit and tomatoes in gently overlapping slices on a large serving plate.

Sprinkle the onion over the slices and season well with salt and pepper. Trickle over the olive oil and any reserved grapefruit juice, and allow the dish to stand at room temperature for about 30 minutes before serving.

FRUIT AND NUT GALETTE

This baked fruit cake is delicious served as a pudding with yoghurt or ice-cream. The quantity given in Apple and Ginger Ice-cream (see next recipe) would be enough to serve 6–8 if you used it as an accompaniment to this dish.

Serves 6–8

8oz (225g) dried apricots, roughly chopped
8oz (225g) dried figs, roughly chopped
1 pear, peeled, cored and chopped
2oz (50g) butter
2oz (50g) brown sugar
1 large egg, beaten
$\frac{1}{4}$ pint (150mls) natural yoghurt
1 teaspoon ground nutmeg
Grated rind and juice of 1 orange
6oz (175g) fresh brown breadcrumbs
4oz (100g) ground almonds
4oz (100g) chopped walnuts or hazelnuts
Fresh fruit and icing sugar (to decorate)

Pre-heat the oven to gas mark 4 (180°C/350°F). Lightly grease a 9-inch (23cm) shallow cake tin and fit a piece of greaseproof paper on to the base. Grease the paper and set aside.

Combine the chopped fruits in a large mixing bowl and add the butter, sugar and egg. Stir in the yoghurt, nutmeg, orange rind and juice. Add the breadcrumbs, and nuts, gently combining them together.

70

Spoon the mixture into the prepared cake tin and bake on the middle shelf in the oven for $1\frac{1}{4}$–$1\frac{1}{2}$ hours, or until a skewer inserted into the centre comes out clean.

To serve: Remove from the oven and allow to cool for 5–10 minutes, then turn the cake out of the tin and remove the greaseproof paper. Decorate with fresh fruit, dust with a little icing sugar and serve warm.

APPLE AND GINGER ICE-CREAM

Serve this ice-cream with Fruit and Nut Galette (see previous recipe), or simply have it on its own or with fresh fruit for a super light dessert.

Serves 4

1lb (450g) cooking apples, peeled and cored
2-inch piece root ginger, peeled and grated
Juice of 1 orange
1 tablespoon honey
1lb (450g) natural yoghurt or fromage frais

Put the apples, ginger and orange juice in a saucepan and cook over medium heat until the apples are soft. Mash the apples until they are smooth, then stir in the honey. Remove from the heat and set aside to cool.

Stir the yoghurt or fromage frais into the cooled apple purée, taste and add extra honey if desired. Spoon the mixture into a freezer tray and freeze until just firm.

YOGHURT FRAPPE

This is as near as you can get to an instant – and totally mouth-watering – dessert. If you want to treat the family as well as yourself, double or quadruple the quantities, depending on the number of hungry mouths you are feeding!

Serves 1

$\frac{1}{4}$ pint (150mls) natural yoghurt
4oz (100g) soft fruit (raspberries, strawberries, blackcurrants, kiwi fruit, blueberries, and so on)
The juice of $\frac{1}{2}$ orange or 2 tablespoons milk
1 sprig of fresh mint, chopped

Liquidise the yoghurt with the fresh fruit, then add enough orange juice or milk to make a soupy consistency. Pour into a small serving bowl and top with the chopped mint. Chill in the refrigerator for about 10–15 minutes before serving.

To serve: Top with chopped seasonal fruits, toasted nuts or desiccated coconut.

71

TOMATO AND SAGE BREAD

This is a very substantial bread, which is particularly good served warm. Sun-dried tomatoes are sold in most delis and some supermarkets these days, but if you can't find them, black or green olives would make a good substitute.

Serves 4

½ sachet easy-blend yeast
8oz (225g) strong plain
white flour
8oz (225g) malted brown flour
1 teaspoon salt
½ pint (300mls) lukewarm milk
2 tablespoons olive oil
1 bunch of sage, roughly chopped
4oz (100g) sun-dried tomatoes,
chopped
1 egg, lightly beaten

Sift the yeast, flours and salt into a large mixing bowl and make a well in the centre. Pour in the milk and olive oil and mix to a soft dough. (Add a small amount of extra flour if the dough is too sticky.) When the dough will leave the sides of the bowl, press it into a ball and tip it out on to a floured surface.

Knead the dough until it is elastic, smooth and shiny (this will take about 10 minutes). Return to the bowl, cover with a piece of lightly greased polythene and put it somewhere warm and draught-free to rise until it has doubled in size.

Knock back the dough, adding the sage and chopped sun-dried tomatoes, kneading them into the dough. Using both of your hands, roll and pat the dough into a round about 10 inches (25cm) in diameter. Place the round on a greased baking sheet and, using a sharp knife, slash the top into a lattice pattern.

Mix the beaten egg with a little salt and water and brush evenly over the loaf to give a good glaze. Return to a warm place and allow to rise again until double in bulk.

Pre-heat the oven to gas mark 6 (200°C/400°F).

Put the bread on the top shelf in the oven and bake for about 30–35 minutes or until it is golden brown (if it browns too quickly, reduce the heat to gas mark 5 (190°C/375°F). The bread is cooked when it sounds hollow when tapped on the bottom; if it doesn't sound hollow when tapped, return it to the oven and continue to cook until it does.

Remove the bread from the oven and cool in the tin for 5 minutes before turning it out on to a wire rack to cool further. Serve warm with, for instance, Cabbage and Walnut (or Hazelnut) Ragout – see the recipe on page 69.

APPLE AND MUSTARD MUFFINS

You can make these savoury muffins in no time at all. Serve them straight from the oven.

Makes 12

4oz (100g) granary flour
4oz (100g) plain flour
¼ teaspoon salt
2½ teaspoons baking powder
2 eggs
3 tablespoons olive oil
1 large dessert apple, cored and grated
1 tablespoon grainy mustard
2oz (50g) cheddar cheese, grated
About 8fl oz (225mls) milk

Pre-heat the oven to gas mark 5 (190°C/375°F) and lightly grease a 12-cup patty tin. Set aside.

Sift the flours, salt and baking powder into a large mixing bowl. Beat together the eggs, olive oil, grated apple, mustard, grated cheese and milk, then add to the flour mixture, stirring quickly together until all the ingredients are combined.

Spoon the mixture into the cups in the greased patty tin (don't bother smoothing the tops) and bake in the oven for 15–20 minutes, or until the muffins are brown and cooked and spring back slightly when pressed with a finger.

Allow to cool slightly, remove from the patty tin and serve at once while they are still warm.

All of the recipes given here are based on the foods recommended on the chart on page 64, so they have the extra plus that while you're enjoying them, you're helping to protect your bones too.

Most of the recipes are for four but don't let that put you off if you normally cook for one or two; you could make the full amount and freeze the extra if you'd rather not have the fiddle of halving or otherwise scaling down the ingredients. And that way you save time and energy another day!

CHAPTER FOUR

THE MENOPAUSE

THE DICTIONARY DEFINES THE MENO-
PAUSE AS THE PERIOD DURING WHICH A
WOMAN'S MENSTRUAL CYCLE ENDS. IT IS
SOMETHING THAT HAPPENS GRADUALLY
(ON AVERAGE IT TAKES ABOUT FOUR
YEARS FROM THE FIRST HOT FLUSH OR
CHANGE IN YOUR MENSTRUAL CYCLE
UNTIL THE TWELVE MONTHS AFTER
YOUR LAST PERIOD WHICH IS USUALLY
REGARDED AS COMPLETION OF THE
PROCESS). IT AFFECTS DIFFERENT
WOMEN IN DIFFERENT WAYS, MANY
WOMEN SCARCELY AT ALL.

In the pages that follow, we look at what the menopause is medically, how it can affect you and your life, and – most importantly – how you can cope with any problems that may arise as you experience it.

WHAT HAPPENS AT THE MENOPAUSE?

To understand what happens to your body at the menopause, you have to go back to the start of your periods.

Your menstrual cycle is part and parcel of your fertility. From the time you are in your middle teens, you produce one or two egg cells each month. These emerge from your ovaries and are swept into one of your Fallopian tubes, which squeezes and pushes them down into the cavity of your womb (uterus is the medical term) – see the illustration below. If intercourse happens at the right time, the sperm cells in your partner's semen swim up into your Fallopian tube and fertilise your egg, which later implants itself into the lining of your womb to grow to maturity. If fertilisation doesn't happen, the egg cells are lost in your vaginal secretions and leave your body during your period.

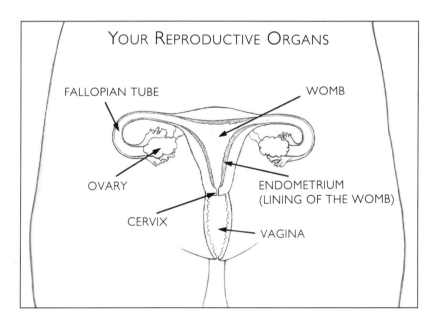

YOUR REPRODUCTIVE ORGANS

FALLOPIAN TUBE

WOMB

OVARY

ENDOMETRIUM
(LINING OF THE WOMB)

CERVIX

VAGINA

As part of the process of producing eggs (called ovulation, medically), your ovaries produce the hormone oestrogen on a rising scale throughout the menstrual cycle – it usually peaks about twelve days after the start of the period, when ovulation takes place. Oestrogen thickens the lining of the womb, called the endometrium. After ovulation, more oestrogen is produced during the second half of the monthly cycle, even if fertilisation doesn't take place, and at this time of the month your ovaries also produce a second hormone called progesterone which works with the oestrogen-thickened lining of your womb to provide a safe nest for your egg. At about the 28th day of your

YOUR OVARIAN HORMONES

OESTROGEN

A hormone is a chemical 'messenger', that is, a chemical which is produced by one part of the body and carried via the blood stream to another some distance away so that it can be active there. Oestrogen is the most important hormone produced by the ovary and is carried to the breasts, womb, bones, skin and brain by your blood vessels.

Oestrogen makes women feminine – it makes breasts grow in young girls, for instance, increases breast size and blood supply in adult women and sometimes makes breasts tender; it thickens and stimulates the lining of the womb and increases its blood supply, making it a safe place for the foetus to grow to maturity. Oestrogen also thickens collagen (the protein network) in skin and bones, and in doing so, gives women protection against osteoporosis and bone fractures. By opposing the action of the 'male' hormones your body produces, such as testosterone, it reduces your risk of heart attack. (Men suffer more heart attacks than women before the age of 50 when both sexes have high levels of hormone; it is women's supply of oestrogen that makes the difference.)

Your body starts producing oestrogen a few years after puberty, increases to its highest output levels when you are cycle if your egg is not fertilised, your level of ovarian hormone production falls dramatically and the lining of your womb is shed – a process called menstruation.

The above cycle occurs each month from a few years after the start of menstruation to the end (menopause). However, as you reach your 40s, you produce eggs less regularly and less frequently, and the rhythm of your monthly hormone production is therefore affected since it's tied to this cycle. This in turn affects your periods – they gradually become scarcer, sometimes heavier, and the two are not mutually exclusive; occasionally they even become *more* frequent than usual.

As you produce eggs more and more rarely, your oestrogen and between about 20 and 40, then falls slightly, although it continues to produce it regularly as part of the fertility cycle. Levels reduce very greatly after the menopause although the hormone doesn't disappear altogether.

PROGESTERONE

Progesterone is the second important hormone produced by the ovaries. It is made by the cells which originally housed your egg and is produced regularly each month by them after the egg is released into your Fallopian tubes. Its major task is to maintain the lining of the womb in good condition and make it 'secretory', that is full of tiny glands which store mucus and control the stimulatory effects of oestrogen. Progesterone also, by changing the pattern of the cells so that your blood vessels narrow, controls and minimises the flow of blood during your period.

Progesterone only appears after ovulation, so women who do not produce eggs do not produce progesterone. Since it is so directly related to the fertility cycle, it reduces after the age of about 45 and stops completely after the menopause. In addition to controlling the effects of oestrogen on the womb and blood flow during menstruation, it can also cause bloating and make you feel sluggish and depressed (premenstrual syndrome).

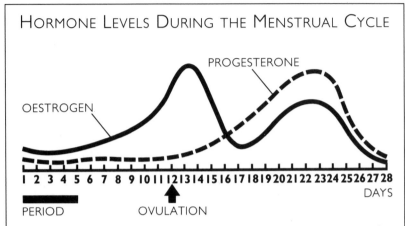

HORMONE LEVELS DURING THE MENSTRUAL CYCLE

PROGESTERONE

OESTROGEN

1 2 3 4 5 6 7 8 9 10 11 12 13 14 15 16 17 18 19 20 21 22 23 24 25 26 27 28
DAYS

PERIOD   OVULATION

Oestrogen levels (the solid black line) peak about 12 days after the start of your period, at ovulation; during the second half of the cycle your body produces **Progesterone** (the broken line) to help your egg survive. After the menopause your body continues to produce oestrogen, but only at about half the lowest rate created during the fertile years (during menstruation).

progesterone levels continue to fall until the progesterone disappears altogether when you stop ovulating. (Your body continues to produce small quantities of oestrogen even after the menopause.) Finally your periods also stop completely.

ARE YOU AT THE MENOPAUSE?

The menopause, medically, is the first day of your last period – although you don't *know* that this is the last period, of course, until about a year later. You can only be sure you have reached the meno-

pause when you've had no bleeding for over a year if you're over 50, over two years if you're under 50.

In terms of age, most women reach the menopause between 50 and 51, although it's quite normal for it to occur across a wider age range, from about 45 to 55, and it's not unusual at any age between 40 and 57. On average, it takes about four years from the first signs and symptoms – usually changes in your menstrual cycle and/or hot flushes – until one year after your last period, when it ends. But 'average' here is extremely variable

78

and can range from the small number of women whose periods may just stop one month, to others who may have irregular periods that start and stop over several years.

The menopause *can* occur earlier than this, although this is unusual. If it comes before the age of 40, it is usually called *premature menopause*, and premature menopause has different implications to normal menopause. It may bring a woman face to face with infertility in a way that a later menopause doesn't, for instance, and also gives rise to more acute worries about health and self image. It can happen for a whole variety of reasons – anorexia is one – and if you believe it may be happening to you, you should consult your doctor.

Apart from age, how can you tell whether *you* are at the menopause? Often it's difficult! Doctors divide the transition period into three main stages which could also act as a guide for you as you go through it:

STAGE 1: PRE-MENOPAUSAL WOMEN, USUALLY IN THEIR EARLY TO MIDDLE 40s, WHO HAVE REGULAR PERIODS. There will be few if any signs of impending menopause at this

stage; it's merely a condition that is kept in mind if other problems occur and you are 'of a certain age'. Some women do suffer occasional hot flushes during the week of their period during this time.

STAGE 2: PERI-MENOPAUSAL WOMEN, USUALLY IN THEIR MIDDLE TO LATE 40s, WHO HAVE MENSTRUATED DURING THE PAST 12 MONTHS BUT WHOSE PERIODS HAVE BECOME IRREGULAR. Indications that you are in this stage are the classic ones usually associated with menopause, namely irregular periods and the onset of flushing. (See pages 83 to 87 for further information on these symptoms.)

STAGE 3: POST-MENOPAUSAL WOMEN, WHO HAVE NOT MENSTRUATED FOR AT LEAST 12 MONTHS. There are relatively few symptoms to guide you at this stage, apart from the obvious one of not having periods, but some women do experience hot flushes now as well as during the previous stage, and vaginal dryness can be a problem. If you aren't sure whether you have reached this stage or not, there is a simple test (it measures hormone levels in the blood) that can confirm or deny it and which is now widely used, especially in detecting the arrival of menopause in women who have had an early hysterectomy (removal of the womb but not the ovaries). Your doctor can arrange for you to have this if there is any doubt.

There are, of course, reasons other than menopause for loss of periods in women between the ages of 40 and 50 – a late pregnancy could be one and other possibilities include coming off the contraceptive pill after you've been using it for a long period of time; some types of hormone injections can also prevent you from having periods. If yours have become irregular or have stopped, and you don't believe that you're entering the menopause, you should consult your doctor to help find out the reason.

IT'S ALWAYS BETTER TO KNOW THE TRUTH THAN TO FEAR THE WORST!

MENSTRUAL CHANGES AT THE MENOPAUSE

For many women the only menstrual 'symptom' they experience during the menopause years is the gradual winding down of their monthly period until it stops; a few don't even have this – one month their period is relatively normal, the next it simply doesn't arrive; nor does it again. For most of us, however, things aren't quite this simple. And, as our reproductive clock goes faster or slower, sudden surges and falls occur in the production of our ovarian hormones, oestrogen and progesterone, which result in changes to our regular bleeding pattern.

What is 'normal'? You can miss the odd period then have another usual or lighter-than-usual one; you can bleed more frequently than before – cycles of 18 days are not uncommon in women in their early 40s; you can have a somewhat heavier-than-before bleed; you can have a shorter or longer span between each period and your period itself can last longer or be shorter. If all of these form a more or less regular and consistent pattern, then they are simply the result of your body preparing itself for the menopause and there is no cause for alarm.

If it's not that easy to figure out what your particular pattern is, try keeping a record of it during this time – you can do this either by marking the days of your period on a menstrual chart like the one below, or on an ordinary calendar or diary. Not only will this help you avoid any 'problem' days as you arrange your life, it could also help your doctor confirm what stage of the menopause you are in, if you have to consult him or her.

Abnormal Bleeding

❝ *My periods are very long, sometimes with only a week clear between them. They start with a brown discharge about a week before the period proper begins.*

I'm spotting all the time. The other night I had a bleed after we had sex and then it tailed off in the morning.

My period was so heavy at work it came through on to my dress and I felt faint. The girls were very good, one of them lent me her coat. I've been taking iron tablets.

There's this pain down below, it gets worse just before a period. My periods are awful, very painful and heavy. I have to go to bed for a day.

My last proper period was two years ago when I was 50. Then I had a year's break. Now I've been bleeding off and on for about ten months. ❞

Very heavy or painful bleeding, or totally irregular or very frequent bleeding, is not normal. If you experience *any* of these or any of the conditions described in the quotes above, you should report

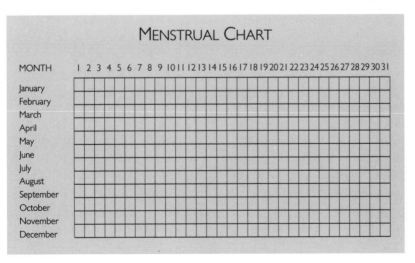

81

them to your doctor. Since there are several possible causes, he or she will probably examine you and perhaps arrange for a specimen to be taken from the lining of your womb so that your particular problem can be identified and treated.

If you turn out to be perfectly healthy (as most women do) you will probably be told you have something called *dysfunctional bleeding*. Dysfunctional bleeding is the name given to any heavy or irregular bleeds which are the result of a mismatch between your oestrogen and progesterone, and is the most common explanation for abnormally heavy or irregular periods that can happen as your reproductive cycle winds down.

The normal hormone release cycle is explained on page 76. Since between the ages of roughly 40 and 50 you produce eggs less regularly, oestrogen thickening of the lining of your womb goes on and on, rather than being controlled and regulated each month by your supply of progesterone, which is only produced when you ovulate. Instead of being shed in its regular way each month by menstruation, therefore, the lining of your

womb is shed only when your oestrogen levels finally fall, and bleeding becomes unpredictable and may be heavy.

Dysfunctional bleeding is easily controlled by progestogens, a chemical substitute for progesterone which works in exactly the same way. You take it from the 11th to the 25th day of the month and about two days after you stop taking it you have a safe, predictable period.

Bleeding after the Menopause

Occasionally after your periods have stopped for a year you can experience bleeding, called *post-menopausal bleeding*. It can be caused by a variety of problems, most of them minor, but you should always report it to your doctor. He or she will probably arrange for a sample to be taken from the lining of your womb to help identify the cause (see page 158). Post-menopausal bleeding can also be treated by progestogen.

Occasionally an investigation uncovers problems which can call for more radical measures such as a hysterectomy (see pages 92 to 94).

The vast majority of women who experience some abnormal

bleeding around this time turn out to have only minor problems that are easily cured. So:

NEVER IGNORE ABNORMAL BLEEDING!

If your periods go on after the age of about 54, by the way, it means that you have higher than usual levels of oestrogen in your body. This is not in itself something to worry about – but you should perhaps tell your doctor when you attend for your three-year cervical smear (see Chapter Five).

OTHER MENOPAUSAL SYMPTOMS

The only specific non-menstrual changes that are clearly associated with the menopause are hot flushes, night sweats and vaginal dryness, although some women also experience emotional ups and downs that are not exclusively to do with the menopause. It is worth stressing here that many women do not suffer any of these conditions and that relatively few are affected by all of them. For those who do experience one or some, however, there are many things that can be done to lessen the problems they cause.

Hot Flushes and Night Sweats

" *Suddenly I feel myself blushing. I can't stop it. It goes on and on, and I feel hot all over my face and neck. It's very embarrassing.*

I have flushes but I just ignore them; they don't really bother me.

Sometimes I wake up and my heart's pounding. Sweat is just pouring off me. I throw off the clothes and go and change.

Sometimes I feel very hot, then I go cold and shivery all over. It's a nuisance – first the central heating is down, then I turn it up again.

I feel hot and cold at times. There's a funny crawly feeling in my arms, like insects crawling under the skin. "

The most common single symptom associated with the menopause is the hot flush – about 80 percent of women experience it at some point. Before the menopause some women do suffer them occasionally but usually only during the week of their period; in the two years following the menopause they can occur more frequently.

Flushes – sometimes called flashes – are harmless, although

they can be a nuisance and a bit embarrassing if circumstances are wrong. You feel hot, and some women blush on their face, neck and breast. They only last a very short time, about a minute or two at most, and can sometimes be followed by a short period of sweating and feeling cold. They are often made worse by stress, anxiety, tension, alcohol, hot drinks and some drugs such as aspirin and vaso-dilators (used to lower blood pressure), and while it's probably not realistic to expect to be able to avoid all of these things all of the time, it helps if you can at least try to minimise your exposure to them if you are prone to flushes.

What Causes Hot Flushes?

Hot flushes occur because certain chemicals are released into your blood system at the time of the menopause. This happens when your oestrogen levels are *falling* only; once your body adjusts to the lower levels, flushes stop. Although flushes are popularly associated with menopausal women, in fact they can occur to most people at some point in their life (think of the stereotypical young man in love who experiences them!) and can even occur in middle-aged women for reasons other than the menopause – those who stop the contraceptive pill, for instance, and women of any age who suddenly stop taking oestrogen therapy (HRT – see Chapter Six).

Whenever it happens, the chemicals being released into your system cause your blood vessels to dilate and so blood rushes to the skin and makes you hot and red. There are literally thousands of intricate blood vessels in your body, so you can imagine how overwhelming the effect of this can be if you do suffer from bad hot flushes.

The body temperature of women changes at the menopause and this can also cause hot flushes (there is a fall of half a degree centigrade in a woman's internal body temperature at this time). This happens because the skin acts as a kind of radiator, and heat is lost from the skin when its tiny blood vessels open and allow more blood to circulate just below the surface. The increased

Hot flushes can be particularly embarrassing if you're out with a colleague – wear layers of clothing if you can and slip off your jacket if you feel one coming on.

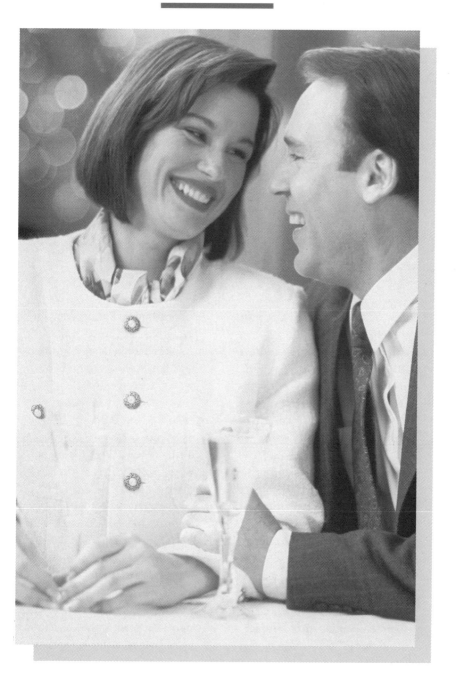

HOW TO BEAT HOT FLUSHES

▲ Take a tepid shower to help you cool down.

▲ Wear several layers of light clothing which you can shed as the temperature rises.

▲ Don't wear a nylon bra – you might be more comforable without one altogether if the weather is hot; otherwise try to wear cotton or some other natural material.

▲ Avoid alcohol, coffee and drugs (such as aspirin and vaso-dilators), which might cause flushing.

flow of blood through the skin sometimes causes dizziness and palpitations but there is no evidence that flushes are harmful, and most women don't feel that they are worth treating – they tend to come and go and disappear after a couple of years. If you feel that your flushes have become too embarrassing to bear, though, you can and should get help to ease the problem. There is a lot your doctor can do to help you, depending on the severity of your symptoms.

You may experience more flushes as the weather gets hotter, but whatever the temperature there are a number of simple basic things you can do to make yourself more comfortable – see the list in the box above.

For more about how to cope with hot flushes and night sweats, see page 164.

Some women find that they experience occasional hot flushes for many years after the menopause, up to 20 years after in extreme cases. The flushes occur for a few days and then disappear for many months. This is because even many years after the menopause, women can go on secreting varying amounts of oestrogen.

When you get hot flushes at night, they can sometimes lead to night sweats, although sweats can

86

occur separately from flushes. Like flushes, night sweats are irritating and uncomfortable rather than dangerous, although they can lead to difficulty in sleeping if they are very frequent. The suggestions given here would work equally well with night sweats.

Vaginal Dryness

66 *I've been meaning to see the doctor for some time but it's a bit embarrassing. You see when we try to have sex it hurts and puts him off. I'm very dry.*

We have started going out together and he's – well, you know – very active. We've been away for the weekend. Anyway, I've come to see if you could give me anything to help – it's a bit difficult. We're thinking of getting married. At our age we need a bit of help. 99

For the vast majority of women, if sex is good before the menopause it's good after. The male hormone, testosterone, is the one that affects your sex drive and this continues to be produced in later life by the ovaries and adrenal glands. However, the vagina is a major user of oestrogen, so as oestrogen levels in your body fall

around menopause, your vaginal walls can become thinner and lose some of their elasticity, and loss of secretions can make your vagina seem dry. This doesn't affect all women, nor does it necessarily affect your sex life – in fact some women find that their sex drive increases as their oestrogen levels fall!

One large study of American women found that those who continued to have sex regularly after the menopause all retained healthily functioning vaginas; in other women, who did not have regular sex, however, the vagina tended to become drier and the lining rather more fragile. Sex then became more difficult. So the motto for sexual function is:

USE IT OR LOSE IT!

Having said that, some women who have very low levels of oestrogen and especially those who have had their womb removed, *can* develop vaginal dryness, and their vaginal opening can become narrow and sore. (About 10 percent of women are believed to suffer from this.) Entry of the penis can be painful and sex becomes unwelcome. You can easily overcome this problem by using oestrogen creams such as Ovestin or Premarin (see page 143), twice a week. Or you can use other lubricants like KY jelly and Replens, which you can buy across the counter, just before intercourse. These latter can be used *instead* of hormone creams or in addition to them.

Emotional Ups and Downs

The menopause has rather a poor image, which is part of a generally negative attitude towards growing older in Western cultures. At least some of what is often put down to menopausal 'moods' is a perfectly healthy antipathy by women to being typecast in this way.

Having said that, some women describe feeling tense and emotional during the time that their hormone levels are changing and there may be a physical base for this. The brain, like the womb, uses the hormone oestrogen and the part that uses it is situated around the thalamus, a region concerned with feelings and emotions. Although doctors do not yet understand enough about oestrogen and the complex changes and fluctuations that happen during the menopausal years, it seems possible that *steep* reductions in the supply of the hormone at that time might result in mood swings and changes. And there is evidence to suggest that some women experience depression after surgical removal of the ovaries, where of course the cut-off of oestrogen is both dramatic and sudden.

❝ *Leading up to the menopause my hormones seemed to be all over the place. I know my body and I felt low at times of the month when before I'd have felt fine.*

I felt so depressed after surgery (hysterectomy and removal of ovaries). I was reasonably prepared for the operation, but afterwards I just felt drained and hadn't much energy. And I went off sex. ❞

If you're feeling anxious, try to talk things over with a friend or counsellor, or consult your general practitioner or practice nurse. Anxiety can make hot flushes and sweats worse and can cause rapid pulse and palpitations, all of which may be made worse by changes in your hormone levels and may be mistakenly taken for purely 'menopausal' symptoms. Anxiety PLUS menopausal symptoms is a very common combination and explains why some women find that their hot flushes do not respond completely to treatment with hormones. If you feel that you are suffering from this combination, seek help: it's there waiting for you!

Other Symptoms

The symptoms dealt with above are the most commonly occurring ones, but there are some others that you can experience, such as joint aches and pains, weight problems, lack of concentration, headaches, nausea, poor memory and irritability. All or most of these are often put down to the menopause when they are found in a woman in her late 40s or early 50s, but in reality most of them are more likely to have other origins (see page 37).

THE SILENT SYMPTOMS

In addition to the visible signs described above, there are two other important things happening to your body at this time that are more difficult to detect but that you need to be aware of. Both can cause potential health problems but the good news is that for both of them prevention is better than cure and prevention has never been easier!

Osteoporosis

Osteoporosis is the name given to the process whereby your bones become 'thinner' and more fragile – a condition that makes you more susceptible to fractures in later life. The hormone oestrogen once again is both the protector and culprit: in your younger days a steady supply helps to keep your bones healthy and reasonably 'dense;' as you approach the menopause and your supply falls, it accelerates a natural thinning process that is already taking place in your body.

Bone thinning, in fact, starts quite early, in your mid-30s, with the loss of about 1 percent of density each year. At the menopause this loss can speed up to about 3 percent per year, although not all women lose this much – there are 'fast' and 'slow' bone losers. Osteoporosis is a common disease in this country and about 20 percent of women currently over 65 suffer from it to one degree or other.

When you are over 65 and are most at risk of fracture, your bone thickness will depend on how fast your bone was lost and how much you had at 35 to 40 – usually called the *peak bone mass*. If as a child you had plenty of

HOW TO PREVENT OSTEOPOROSIS

▲ Have enough calcium in your diet

▲ Make sure you have reasonable exposure to sunlight, which produces vitamin D in the skin (in moderation only, obviously – see page 111 for guidance)

▲ Take regular weight-bearing exercise like walking (see page 56)

▲ Don't smoke.

calcium in your diet (see page 64 for a listing of calcium-rich foods), you have exercised sensibly and regularly throughout your life and are a non-smoker, you'll probably still have dense bones in middle age. On the other hand, if you are a heavy smoker, or if you missed periods regularly because of marathon running, fanatical slimming or anorexia, you may well have fragile bones.

If you're worried (or curious!) about what *your* bone density is, you can take a test to find out. If your doctor feels you are at risk, he or she may well suggest that you go on HRT to prevent further density loss. Taking HRT will reduce the amount of loss immediately, just like turning off a tap, and the effect will last as long as you continue to take it – although no one yet knows how long the protection lasts after you stop the treatment. Several large studies have shown a 50 percent reduction in fractures in women who have taken HRT for five to six years.

There are other factors besides HRT, however, that are important in preserving bone density – see the box above.

See pages 100 to 102 for more about osteoporosis and how to prevent it.

Coronary Heart Disease
Coronary heart disease occurs when the arteries that carry blood to the heart muscle narrow, and oxygen from the blood can't reach

the muscle in sufficient quantities to keep the heart functioning efficiently.

The heart lets you know when this is happening by anginal pain, the pain that occurs when the muscle 'complains' about the lack of oxygen. You will feel the pain first in your chest or upper stomach although it may also spread to your neck or arm; it's most likely to happen when the heart is working hardest, pumping blood to the stomach after a heavy meal or during exercise.

A blood clot can also block the coronary artery. When this happens, part of the heart muscle expires and you have what is called a heart 'attack'.

The arteries carrying blood to your heart can narrow because they become furred up with fat (a condition known as atheroma) – the result is that insufficient oxygen reaches your heart to keep it functioning efficiently.

Heart disease is more frequent during and after the menopause than before because clotting factors and fats in your blood increase as oestrogen levels fall. A woman of 45 who has had the menopause is therefore more likely to have a heart attack than a woman of 55 who is still menstruating.

As with osteoporosis, there is a whole host of preventive measures you can take that will lessen your particular risk considerably – see the box below. Distribution of body fat also plays its part in who runs more risk of heart

HOW TO PREVENT HEART DISEASE

▲ Switch to a healthy diet, and in particular eat less animal fat and more fibre

▲ Exercise regularly, particularly aerobic exercise such as swimming, cycling and running

▲ Don't smoke and cut down on heavy drinking

▲ Taking HRT may substantially reduce your risk of heart disease.

disease. For more on this and how to prevent heart disease, see Chapter Five.

SURGICAL MENOPAUSE

About 12 percent of British women have a surgical menopause rather than a natural one, usually as a last-resort cure for excessively heavy bleeding or to remove fibroids (lumps of muscle that cause pain and bleeding) from their womb. Although a hysterectomy is regarded as major stomach surgery, it is a safe procedure these days and need not be a worrying thing to contemplate. There are two different types of surgical menopause:

HYSTERECTOMY WITH CONSERVATION OF THE OVARIES – that is the womb only is removed. If you have this operation, you will not have periods afterwards although your 'true' menopause will not take place until the usual age, around 50; a small proportion of women who have this operation do reach it earlier than normal. You will probably have a few flushes immediately after the operation, and when 'true' menopause occurs hot flushes and night sweats might be bothersome. Since it's particularly diffi-

cult in this case to know if you *have* definitely reached menopause, your doctor can confirm it by administering a simple blood test (see page 79). HRT (hormone replacement therapy) may be recommended at this time since it gives some protection against flushes and also osteoporosis.

HYSTERECTOMY WITH REMOVAL OF BOTH OVARIES – this type of hysterectomy causes instant menopause. It is usually carried out if your surgeon has reason to believe that you have serious problems such as ovarian cysts. Hot flushes and sweats can be more severe after this operation and sometimes depression and loss of sex drive may occur, particularly in younger women. HRT is always prescribed for patients after this type of hysterectomy unless there's a good reason not to give it (see page 133). If HRT is not used there is an increased risk of osteoporosis, fractures and coronary heart disease. Removal of one ovary does not cause instant menopause.

Hysterectomies can be performed via the lower belly, when you are left with a (hopefully neat!) incision just above your

SURGICAL MENOPAUSE

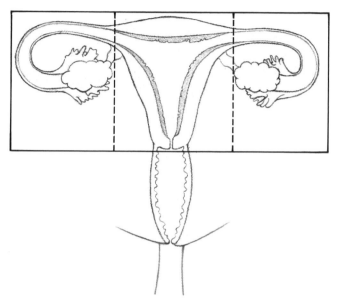

The outer lines show what is removed when you have a hysterectomy *with* removal of both ovaries and Fallopian tubes; the inner, broken, lines show the less radical version, where only the womb itself is removed.

pubic area or through the vagina. You will be required to go into hospital to have a hysterectomy and will stay there for an average of about seven to ten days; the operation itself takes about $1\frac{1}{2}$ hours. Recovery is reasonably slow and on average it takes about three months before you are functioning normally again. There is now a possible third option for women who suffer from heavy bleeding, to have an *endometrial ablation* – removal of the lining of the womb by laser surgery. This is a new operation which is still being developed, but it offers a much less radical cure for excessively heavy bleeding than hysterectomy; patients stay in hospital for only one night and the usual recovery time is about one week. Your periods will stop after this operation but true menopause will not occur until the usual age. If you take HRT after this operation you still need to use progestogen supplements (see page 140) as small pockets of womb lining may be left behind.

A Final Word

If you asked a doctor to draw a graph of what happens at the menopause, he or she might create something like the chart below.

It would be fair to say that the chart tends to be a collection of *problems* experienced by millions of women all over the world between the ages of 40 and 65. But doctors tend to see women who have problems rather than those who don't, and their view of the menopause is coloured by their experience of women as

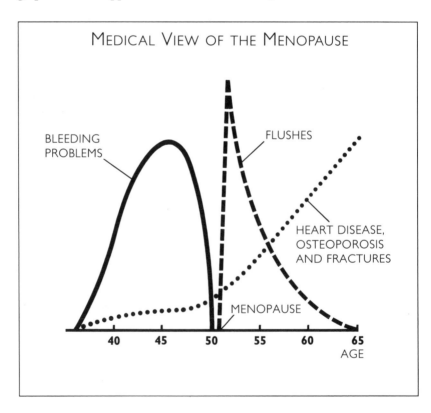

MEDICAL VIEW OF THE MENOPAUSE

BLEEDING PROBLEMS

FLUSHES

HEART DISEASE, OSTEOPOROSIS AND FRACTURES

MENOPAUSE

40   45   50   55   60   65
AGE

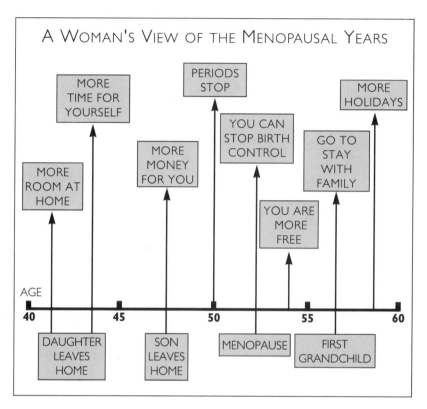

A WOMAN'S VIEW OF THE MENOPAUSAL YEARS

MORE TIME FOR YOURSELF

PERIODS STOP

MORE HOLIDAYS

YOU CAN STOP BIRTH CONTROL

GO TO STAY WITH FAMILY

MORE MONEY FOR YOU

MORE ROOM AT HOME

YOU ARE MORE FREE

AGE

40   45   50   55   60

DAUGHTER LEAVES HOME

SON LEAVES HOME

MENOPAUSE

FIRST GRANDCHILD

'patients' (that is, people complaining of various symptoms such as flushes or vaginal problems, and asking for help to cure them).

There is another way to look at it, and that is from your point of view. You will have quite a different perspective on how things are going, and it is sometimes worth spelling out the positive things that happen during this changing part of your life, as one of the authors has done above for *her* life. We hope your view of your circumstances is equally positive!

Your last period truly is only another date in your life. It is of no importance in itself but it can be a useful point in time for you to remember to take care of yourself and to start to make the most of the thirty years or so of life that lies ahead of you.

95

CHAPTER FIVE

LOOKING AFTER YOUR HEALTH

WILL YOUR HEALTH CHANGE
DURING AND AFTER THE MENO-
PAUSE? THE MENOPAUSE ITSELF
WILL NOT USUALLY AFFECT YOUR
GENERAL HEALTH, EXCLUDING IRRE-
GULAR PERIODS AND HOT FLUSHES,
SO IF YOU WERE HEALTHY BEFORE
YOU SHOULD REMAIN HEALTHY
DURING AND AFTER IT.

Some women, in fact, feel much fitter after the menopause – especially if they have suffered more than usually from irregular and heavier periods and more-severe-than-usual flushes. Many report a real surge in energy and vitality levels; in fact, it's not hard to find examples of such women in public life as we look around us!

What is beyond dispute is that staying healthy does take a little more effort as you get older, so you may have to work harder to keep your body as fit as it was when you were 25. If you do, though, the results are quick to appear and it's well worth it.

MAINTAINING GOOD HEALTH

If your lifestyle is a healthy one, reasonably free from stress and you are happy, your life will not only be better, the odds are that it will be longer too. And while there are some aspects of our lives that are difficult or impossible to change (our physical environment is often one, the height we grow to another), there are things we can do for ourselves and our families that can have an important bearing on our current and future health. The two obvious examples are to follow a good diet and to exercise, both now proved to be key factors in preventing or minimising the effects of many diseases that we become vulnerable to as we grow older, such as heart attack, osteoporosis, stroke and some cancers.

What *is* a good diet? In Chapter Three of this book we have spelled out the kind of diet that will help you prepare well for the menopause. As you reach the menopause and go beyond it, it becomes even more important to adopt healthy eating habits – so turn back to page 62 and look again at our pre-menopause diet guidelines, and make sure you continue with them not only then but during your menopause and after it too.

Watching your Weight

❝ *I despair of ever looking slim again. I've tried diet after diet – and nothing happens. I'm beginning to believe there's something in that old wives' tale about middle-aged women having to be plump!*

I'm not really fat – but I did feel bunched up all the time and wished I could look better in clothes. So I started doing these stretching exercises for my tummy and they seem to have helped a lot.

I get really depressed when I turn on the TV and see all these sylph-like young women advertising things. Why can't we go back to all those Rubens ladies that the Victorians were so fond of?

I hate diets! So I've decided to keep fit to feel healthy – I'm still a couple of pounds heavier than I was when I was younger, but I feel and look better than I did before. 〃

The first thing to admit when you're over 40 is that you're probably never going to be the same shape as you were when you were 20. As we mature we burn up calories more slowly, with the result that even a fairly modest amount of food can start putting weight on us rather than maintaining our size as it did when we were younger.

There are simple things we can do to keep our weight in check, though – watching what we eat is one, and we are lucky because the types of food we should eat to stay healthy are generally those that are least fattening. Taking regular exercise also helps: it increases our metabolism (which is what burns up those calories) with the result that our body 'gets through' food more quickly. Since exercise, too, helps cut

down our risks of many diseases and illnesses, it makes sense to include some in your daily life from all points of view.

Having said all that, you needn't be paranoid about putting on a few extra pounds from a health viewpoint. Your *shape*, in fact, is more important than your weight providing you're not in the obese band in the chart on the opposite page.

Women's magazines wax on eloquently about us being shaped like apples and pears – well, there's a medical precedent for this. Men, on the whole, are shaped like apples: when they put on weight they tend to put it on around their middle, increasing the ratio of their waist to hip measurement; women usually put fat on around the hips and thighs (the traditional pear), which can leave them with a nice neat waist and a hip size they lie about whenever possible! There are, however, women who put on weight according to the 'apple' pattern and if you're one of them, you need to be more careful about gaining weight than pear-shaped women; the 'apple' pattern is known to expose you to a higher risk of developing heart disease.

HEIGHT AND WEIGHT CHART

HEIGHT	SENSIBLE WEIGHT	SLIGHTLY FAT	OBESE
5ft 0in	7st 0lb – 8st 13lb	9st 2lb – 10st 8lb	10st 10lb+
1in	7st 2lb – 9st 0lb	9st 6lb – 10st 13lb	11st 4lb+
2in	7st 6lb – 9st 4lb	9st 10lb – 11st 4lb	11st 10lb+
3in	7st 9lb – 9st 8lb	10st 1lb – 11st 9lb	12st +
4in	7st 12lb – 10st 0lb	10st 5lb – 12st 1lb	12st 4lb+
5in	8st 2lb – 10st 4lb	10st 10lb – 12st 6lb	12st 10lb+
6in	8st 6lb – 10st 8lb	11st 1lb – 12st 11lb	13st 2lb+
7in	8st 9lb – 10st 13lb	11st 5lb – 13st 3lb	13st 9lb+
8in	8st 13lb – 11st 4lb	11st 11lb – 13st 8lb	14st 1lb+
9in	9st 2lb – 11st 8lb	12st 1lb – 14st 0lb	14st 7lb+
10in	9st 6lb – 11st 13lb	12st 6lb – 14st 6lb	14st 11lb+
11in	9st 10lb – 12st 4lb	12st 11lb – 14st 12lb	15st 5lb+
6ft 0in	10st 0lb – 12st 9lb	13st 2lb – 15st 3lb	15st 11lb+
1in	10st 4lb – 13st 0lb	13st 7lb – 15st 9lb	16st 3lb+
2in	10st 8lb – 13st 4lb	13st 12lb – 16st 1lb	16st 9lb+

Note: The above weights are *with* clothes; deduct 4lb if you weigh yourself without clothes. Heights are measurement without shoes.

If you find yourself in the band marked obese in our table, you should try as hard as you can to cut down your weight – when you're carrying around this amount of excess you're more prone to heart attack and stroke than slimmer women. If you find that it's too hard to do this on your own, go to your doctor for help.

You can, of course, be too *thin* and this, too, can give you health problems – very thin women are more likely to suffer from osteoporosis than their plumper sisters. So watch out if you're way *under* weight, and try to put some on!

Most of us will be somewhere between these two extremes, perhaps feeling a bit too plump and wishing vaguely that we were a bit thinner. Obviously it's important to feel good about yourself and if feeling that you're too fat is preventing that, then you should do something about it. But ask yourself honestly if it's all that important to your sense of happiness and well-being: being slim is being girlish; being a little rounder is being womanly.

CUTTING DOWN THE RISKS OF OSTEOPOROSIS AND HEART DISEASE

As we have already seen in Chapter Four, two 'silent' effects of the menopause are an increased risk of developing the bone thinning disease osteoporosis and a greater vulnerability to different types of heart disease.

Osteoporosis

Osteoporosis causes many different types of fracture in later life, one of the most serious being fracture of the hip – and there are about 46,000 of those per year in England and Wales among older people.

Who is most at risk? Research suggests that you are more likely to get osteoporosis if you:

△ are a woman

△ reach your menopause early (ie before 45)

△ smoke regularly

△ are white or oriental

△ are too thin (see page 99)

CHUSE To Prevent Osteoporosis

CALCIUM Eat more (at least 800mg daily)

HORMONES Try them – ask your doctor

ULTRA VIOLET Sunlight: 15 minutes daily outdoors

SMOKING Cut down or Stop!

EXERCISE Get going

A HEALTHY BONE

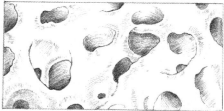

B OSTEOPOROTIC BONE

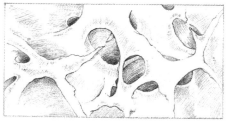

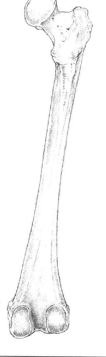

In illustration (**A**) above the bone is still healthy but by (**B**) the amount of calcium and protein inside the bone is already reduced and the bone is becoming 'thin'. Once bones become fragile, they are more prone to fracture.

△ don't have enough calcium in your diet (see page 64 for a list of calcium-rich foods)

△ don't exercise

△ have a family history of osteoporosis

△ take corticosteroids (prescribed for asthma or joint pains) or thyroxine (for thyroid disease).

Whether this list is relevant to you or not, there are many simple things you should do to cut down your risk of developing osteoporosis – see pages 89 to 90 for more information; the box on the left might help too. And since *falling* is usually the event that causes a fracture, it makes sense to take a few precautions against this as well – for instance, make sure that your stairs are well lit and that there are no loose rugs or slippery floors around. ABOVE ALL

If you are very worried about the health of your bones, ask your doctor to arrange a Bone Density Test, which will tell you how much bone loss you've suffered. If there has been more than average, he or she will probably recommend that you take HRT unless there's a good reason for you not to.

Heart Disease

Heart disease is often regarded as something that affects men rather than women, but about 66,000 women, most of them over the age of 50, die of it each year in England and Wales. Heart disease and its causes are covered in detail on pages 90 to 92.

Some of the causes of heart disease go back to our childhood or before – even the nourishment given to a foetus in the womb can affect its blood pressure and risk of heart disease 50 years later – but there is a lot you can do to minimise your chances of getting this disease.

You are most at risk if you:

△ have a family history of heart disease

△ smoke cigarettes

△ are male

△ are over 60 if you are a woman, 50 if you are a man

△ suffer from high cholesterol

△ have high blood pressure (hypertension)

△ suffer from diabetes (see page 113)

△ are obese (see chart on page 99).

It's impossible to stress too strongly the effect smoking has on your general health and well-being but where heart disease is concerned the risk is very specific: if you are a smoker under the age of 45 you have *14 times* the normal risk of heart attack. And the earlier you stop the better: although it helps if you stop at

Exercise helps prevent heart disease and makes you feel better too.

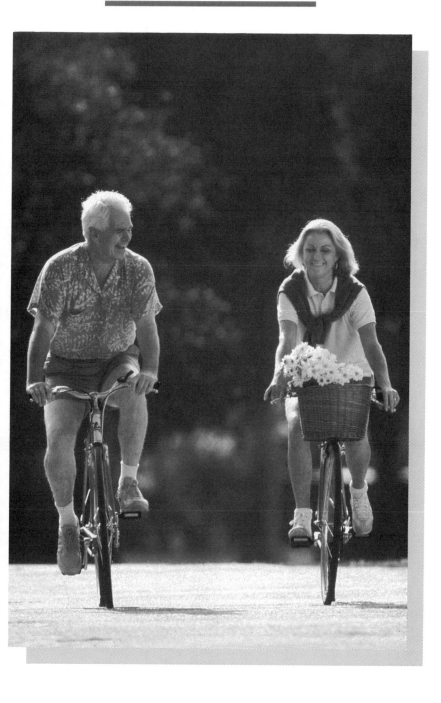

any age, research shows that stopping after 60 is less beneficial than stopping at 30.

There are advantages to being a woman where heart attacks are concerned, and you are much less likely than a man to die of one at a young age – as you can see, our incidence of heart attack is roughly ten years behind that of men.

A high level of cholesterol in your blood can narrow the arteries through which blood flows to your heart – thus causing a heart attack. Women are much more resistant to high cholesterol than men but even so this is something you should keep tabs on as time goes by. You can get a cholesterol level test from your doctor, and some well-woman clinics and health-check programmes also do them.

If you find you have high cholesterol (usually 7.0–7.5mmol/1 is considered the level at which you need treatment) you will probably need to go on a cholesterol-lowering diet. The main recommendations of such a diet are to:

△ reduce animal fat intake by cutting down on rich dairy products and meat

△ use a polyunsaturated spread instead of butter

△ eat a maximum of two egg yolks per week

△ avoid foods rich in cholesterol such as liver, kidney, shrimps and prawns

△ increase your fibre intake by eating more fruit, oat cereals, peas and green beans

To help your heart (although it doesn't decrease your cholesterol):

△ eat at least three oily fish meals (salmon, trout, mackerel, herring) a week instead of meat

△ make sure you have enough Vitamin C (from fresh vegetables and fresh fruit juices).

Our blood pressure varies all the time – it goes up when we're exercising, experiencing strong emotion or having sex and falls when we're asleep. But there are acceptable levels within which this variation occurs and if your blood pressure is consistently higher than it should be for your age, it can be a warning of an increased risk of stroke and heart disease. Your doctor is probably already monitoring your blood pressure – but if this isn't happening, you should try to make sure that he or she does next time you visit.

If you do suffer from high blood pressure, cut down on the amount of salt you take, drink less alcohol and eat healthily (see our guidlines on page 62); yoga and relaxation exercises can also help. Reducing your blood pressure to normal levels is well worth it even if you have to stick with treatment for the rest of your life; by doing so, you'll reduce your risk of stroke by half.

BEATING BREAST CANCER

Most women have problems with their breasts from time to time but most of these problems have nothing to do with breast cancer: your breasts can be too small or too large, one can be larger than the other (it nearly always is) and so on. Breast pain is very common, too, particularly the week before your period starts and during the first few months of HRT treatment. If such pain is containable it's best to leave it as is; if it is *very* painful, your doctor can help – the antihor-

mone Danazol is sometimes prescribed, for instance, although it stops your periods.

A surprising amount of minor breast pain is caused by ill-fitting bras made of artificial fabrics. If you suspect this may be the cause of your discomfort, then switch to cotton and try a size larger than your usual one – you'd be surprised at how often this works!

Lumps in your breast are also quite common – and it's important to stress that nine out of ten of them are benign and will cause you no trouble at all. However, lumps *can* be a sign of cancer and it's important, therefore, that if you find one you report it to your doctor. Cancer of the breast is, unfortunately, still all too common among women in this country – about one in twelve of us will contract it at some point in our lives, and it is the commonest cause of death for pre-menopausal women.

Although there are as yet no clear guidelines about how to prevent breast cancer, there is now evidence of who is at most risk. You are at risk if:

△ your mother or sister has suffered from it

△ you started your periods at an early age and have your menopause late (probably because your exposure to oestrogen is longer than usual)

△ you are childless

△ you have a poor diet, especially one that is high in cholesterol and low in fibre

ALL of us – whether we qualify as being at risk or not – should help minimise the risks of this cancer by checking our breasts about once a month, preferably the week after our period if we are still menstruating (check at a regular time each month if you're not). This should enable us to spot any lumps when they first appear, so that they can be dealt with sooner rather than later. (See the box opposite for how to check your breasts.)

Make Time for a Mammogram

66 *I went to have my breasts X-rayed thinking it would be quite gentle and quick. It wasn't! The radiographer manhandled first one breast then the other between these two plates and sort of squashed them together until I could hardly bear it.*

I absolutely panicked when I found the lump on my breast. But I got it checked out and it was okay. It was such a relief. . . 99

A more accurate method of detecting breast cancer is mammography. A mammogram is a sort of X-ray (your breasts are squeezed, one by one, between two plates and photographed) which can detect any shadows or spots in your breasts at a very early stage. It is now offered FREE to every woman over 50 in this country every three years. If you have a family history of breast cancer you can get regular free mammograms under this age, and if you are over 64 you can have the test on request. If you decide to have HRT your doctor may suggest that you have a mammogram before you start to take it.

If you are registered with a doctor and are of the right age you should be having a mammogram automatically every three years; if you aren't, make sure that you are put on your doctor's register – there is a lot of evidence to show that having

FIRST LOOK

▲ Stand in front of a long mirror in good light and undress to the waist.

▲ Keep your arms at your sides and look at your breasts from every angle – including *under them.*

▲ Now lift your arms above your head and check for any discolouring or rashing around your nipples.

▲ Raise then lower your arms sideways; watch for unusual shapes or movements while you do it.

▲ Put your hands on your hips; your skin shouldn't ruck as you do it and your breasts should move smoothly.

THEN FEEL

▲ Check your nipples for discharge by squeezing them gently.

▲ Using your fingers, work gently outwards in small circular motions until you've covered both breasts (including underneath).

▲ Put one arm then the other above your head (bend your elbow while you do it), then check that breast to make sure there are no hard lumps on it.

▲ Finally, raise each arm in turn again and feel for lumps around the breast/armpit area.

this test regularly is a very good way of finding any problems at a very early stage and treating them successfully.

If you do find a lump and it is diagnosed as being malignant (that is, cancerous) you needn't despair. If your cancer is found early, there is a 90 percent chance of complete cure – a much better rate than most other cancers.

Early breast cancer is usually treated (depending on the size of the lump) either by removing the lump from your breast (called

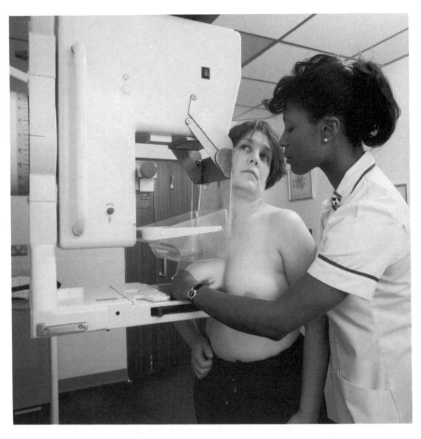

Mammograms only take a few minutes – and they can save you years of pain.

lumpectomy) or by removing part of the breast itself if the lump has 'spread' or is quite large. Occasionally, if discovery is later than wished, it's necessary to remove the entire breast (mastectomy); however, with better and more regular screening, this is happily becoming a rarer operation these days. After the operation, you'll be given che-motherapy or X-ray treatment to make sure that there will be no recurrence of the cancer, and you'll continue to be checked at regular intervals for several years until everyone is absolutely certain you're in the clear.

108

Tamoxifen is one highly successful drug treatment for breast cancer and is often given to women after they have been operated on. Since it's an anti-oestrogen, it may give you hot flushes, although it does increase bone strength so helps you in the fight against osteoporosis. Researchers believe there is a possibility that this drug may be effective in *preventing* breast cancer among high-risk women, and a large-scale research project is now in progress to test this.

PREVENTING OTHER CANCERS

Although breast cancer is the most common cancer found in women, particularly older ones, sadly as we grow older we are susceptible to other types as well. Again, however, there is a lot we can do to prevent or minimise the effects of these diseases.

Cervical cancer is relatively common – women who smoke and are sexually active are most at risk – and nearly 2000 people a year die from it in England and Wales. The good news is that this death rate is falling every year because the disease is eminently treatable if it's caught early, and it's increasingly being caught early because the

cervical 'smear' test is now very widely available.

The 'smear' test couldn't be simpler: your doctor or nurse inserts a metal speculum into your vagina to get a clear view of the area, then scrapes some sample cells from the cervix and smears them on to a slide, which is then analysed for any irregularities. This test has an excellent detection record and an early diagnosis radically improves your chances of cure.

❝ I was really quite worried by my (smear) test. I don't like having internal examinations and this sort of cancer is scary. But actually in the end it wasn't as bad as I'd expected and it only lasted a minute or so.

The worst thing for me was the way I was given the results. I didn't know what 'minor inflammation' meant, and until I talked to my doctor I was convinced it was cancer.

I always have my smear test every three years. It's reassuring for me to know that everything's fine. Once I did have an infection which showed up on the test, but it was treated straight away. ❞

Sometimes the test shows up what are called false positives

– so don't be alarmed if you're recalled for a second smear. What happens is that the test checks *pre-cancerous* cells and any changes (including those created by infections) show up, whether they're cancerous or not. If anything at all shows up in the first test, you're recalled for a second, more specific one, which will monitor and 'explain' the findings of the first. If you're worried or have any doubts, don't hesitate to ask your doctor to explain your results in detail; all anxieties are lessened considerably by accurate information.

If you have been sexually active and you have not had a hysterectomy, you can have a smear test free at regular intervals on the national health – make sure you do!

Ovarian cancer is more difficult to treat than either breast or cervical cancer and it causes about 4000 deaths per year in this country. Again, however, if it is detected early, the prognosis for recovery is good. Unfortunately it's less easy than some other cancers to spot (your ovaries are hidden in your pelvis and changes can be difficult to see) but a vaginal ultrasound test has recently been developed that is showing good results, so this may be changing. (An ultrasound is an instrument probably more often associated with picturing your baby when it's a foetus in your womb, but it's also used to scan and check the state of your pelvic organs generally.)

If you are bleeding irregularly (see page 81), don't ignore it – go to your doctor and have it checked. It *could* be the first sign of an ovarian cancer.

Bowel cancer is equally common in both sexes and the incidence does increase a bit as you get older, so it's worth being extra careful here too.

If you've noticed a recent change in your bowel movements, or if you are bleeding from the rectum, see your doctor: both need investigation.

Lung Cancer This used to be considered a male disease but it is more common among women than it used to be and now causes about 10,000 deaths a year in England and Wales. The causes of lung cancer are clear and unequivocal and prevention can be summed up in two words:

DON'T SMOKE

Melanoma is the word used to describe cancer of the skin – still comparatively rare in the United Kingdom but it does occur. It is commoner in very fair people (those with very pale skin and freckles are particularly at risk) who are exposed to sunlight, but it can, in fact, occur anywhere on the body and not necessarily on exposed parts. One symptom is a brown or black wart that enlarges or bleeds or itches.

Melanoma can be prevented if you use a barrier cream before you sunbathe (6 plus is necessary for fair-skinned people in Mediterranean-type sunlight) and if you limit your exposure to less than an hour a day. You don't need to don a swimming costume and point your whole body towards the sun to get enough

vitamin D, by the way; if you expose your face and hands for the amount of time suggested above, you'll get enough to protect your whole body.

MINIMISING OTHER PROBLEMS

Joint Pains
Joint pains and stiffening of the muscles are common after physical exercise at any age, and usually pass off quickly; general stiffening of the muscles is something that can happen to many people as they grow older (although if you adopt a more active lifestyle you'll get less of it in the first place). But stiffening may also be caused by arthritis, a disease that causes swelling and inflammation in our joints, and in this case you will need treatment to help it; women's joint pains are *not* caused by the menopause, although there's a common belief that some of them are – there's even a type of swollen fingers which is mistakenly called menopausal arthritis.

There are two types of arthritis that occur in middle-aged and older women. *Osteoarthritis* is often the result of damage to the

111

joint by an early accident or hard physical labour. It can affect any joint but is particularly common in weight-bearing joints like hips and knees. Chemical changes occur in the cartilage surface (cartilage is the name given to the gristle at the end of each bone) and are signalled by acute pain and swelling of the joints themselves; these wear off eventually and the illness then enters its chronic phase when, ironically, it may be pain-free. Osteoarthritis has nothing to do with osteoporosis (except that they both affect bones).

Rheumatoid arthritis affects the lining of the joints first and causes stiffness, swelling and deformity. There is now a blood test that can discover whether you have rheumatoid arthritis or not, and you should arrange to have it if you think you might have this disease.

There are many available treatments for arthritis – exercise can help, for instance (swimming is particularly good) and fish oil can help minor, milder types. For more severe sufferers recent advances in joint replacement surgery can revolutionise their lives; hip and knee replacements are now very common, and tendon operations are also on the increase these days.

You can help prevent arthritis by avoiding lifting heavy objects, especially with a bent back; by investing in cupboards above waist height so that you stretch (although not too much) rather than bend, high chairs and a comfortable bed. And keep your back straight!

Thyroid Problems

The thyroid gland in our neck produces a hormone (called thyroxine) which controls the rate at which our body burns up calories. As we become older it usually functions more slowly although there is a range within which it is considered to be working normally. Sometimes, however, thyroids become overactive – common signs are extreme thinness, tremulousness and protruding eyes; the heart rate can increase and sometimes diarrhoea is also present. The reverse condition also happens: the symptoms here are tiredness, weight gain, constipation, feeling cold and sluggish – and there may also be some emotional changes and problems. An underactive thyroid can sometimes lead to heart trouble since it can cause fat to build up in the coronary arteries.

Both of these conditions can be diagnosed by blood test and controlled with tablets. If you have any reason to suspect you might have an over-active or under-active thyroid you should consult your doctor so that you can start treatment.

Diabetes

Diabetes, a condition in which the body fails to cope efficiently with sugar, is one of the commonest health problems in this country and affects 2 percent of the population.

There are two major types of diabetes; one, which mainly affects younger people, is caused by a lack of insulin and the other, whose cause is unknown, which affects mostly middle-aged and elderly people. Symptoms of mature diabetes include thirst, a frequent need to urinate, weight gain and genital itch. Diabetes

can greatly increase your risk of heart disease and stroke, so it's particularly important to control your diet and weight if you are diabetic. Your doctor can help you with diet sheets if you need them – a diabetic diet is very similar to the general healthy heart diet guidelines we have given on page 62. HRT may help you reach a suitable cholesterol level, which could help cut the risks somewhat.

AVOIDING PREGNANCY

❝ My periods are getting scarcer and scarcer now – I'm nearly 50. Do I need to bother with birth control?

I've taken the pill for nearly 20 years – do I have to keep using it even during the menopause?

I don't like the bother of contraception any more and I don't want more kids, should I be sterilised?

Will the pill help my hot flushes? ❞

Most women in their 40s, given a straight choice, would choose *not* to become pregnant, yet nearly half the women in this age group do not use birth control on a regular basis, and there are many unplanned pregnancies among women over 40.

Why does this happen? Most likely because many older women realise that it's much less likely that they'll get pregnant than a younger woman. This is probably true, particularly as you progress into your 40s, but women as old as 50 have become pregnant and it's not at all uncommon to conceive in your early to mid-40s. Even though we do produce fewer eggs as we get older, most of us continue to produce a few right up until the menopause – and you only need to fertilise one to have a baby!

For peace of mind, therefore, and also to aid your general health and well-being (older women usually have a more difficult time during pregnancy than younger ones), you should continue to use birth control until at least a year after the menopause, or two years if you're under 50. If you are using a method now, and are happy with it, there is no reason why you should change – just keep on using it regularly and carefully. If, for some reason, you have stopped taking precautions and want to restart, or if you are considering starting, there are some

points to bear in mind as you make your choice.

The Pill

The pill remains the easiest-to-use form of contraception there is – if you're confident that you can remember to take it regularly! It is also the most *effective* form of contraception so far invented. Contrary to rumour, it is completely safe to continue taking it after the age of 40; there was a scare about increased risks for older women a few years ago but it's now recognised that this only applies to women who smoke. During the early years of the pill, each tablet contained quite a high dose of oestrogen; nowadays it's recognised that this isn't necessary so all the pills currently on the market have much lower amounts.

If you smoke you run a greater risk of heart disease and because of this, most doctors advise you to switch to some other form of contraception after the age of about 35. (You may be able to take a progestogen-only pill, however, see page 115).

Using the pill at any age will give you increased protection against some common female problems and since the incidence of these problems tends to increase with age, the pill can play its part in maintaining your health during your 40s. The pill:

△ protects against heavy bleeding (it imposes a regular, controlled pattern)

△ protects against cysts and ovarian cancer (it halves the risk)

△ protects against endometrial cancer (cancer of the lining of the womb) (it halves the risk)

△ reduces the likelihood of breast lumps

△ helps prevent osteoporosis

△ eliminates hot flushes (in most women).

The pill will *not* protect you against cervical or breast cancer (but it won't increase your risk of getting these illnesses either), nor does it offer any protection against heart disease or stroke.

If you continue to take the pill after 40, make sure that your doctor is aware of it and that he or she monitors your blood pressure regularly. If you experience very severe headaches, speech dis-turbance, loss of vision, one-sided numbness, sudden severe pains in your chest, painful swelling in the calf of your leg, or if you cough up blood-stained phlegm, you should go to see your doctor; he or she will probably recommend that you use a different form of birth control.

Although most types of contraceptive pill contain both oestrogen and progestogen (an artificial form of the natural hormone progesterone), there is a progestogen-only pill available these days which, if taken regularly at the same time every day, has a good safety record. Some smokers can take this pill, although most over-35s who smoke switch to non-oral types of birth control. Where there is a choice, it is better to stay on an oestrogen plus progestogen pill; progestogen only ones will not protect you against menopausal hot flushes.

If you take the pill around the time of the menopause, you won't suffer from irregular periods since the pill will regularise them for you. However, it will make it more difficult for you to tell when your menopause is starting – and finishing. If this becomes a problem for you,

115

discuss it with your doctor; he or she will probably recommend that you use another, 'barrier' method of contraception such as the diaphragm or sheath for three or four months so that you can check the situation.

IUDS (Intra-uterine Devices)

An IUD is a small coil-like device which is put into your womb (usually by a doctor) and which prevents a fertilised egg implanting itself. Once it has been inserted it remains there – until you need to change it (they usually last about seven years). It's very safe and comfortable to wear, and there are no added hazards in using it over the age of 40. You should keep your IUD in place for about a year after you reach the menopause. Then it should be removed.

IUDs are fine for most people, but if you have a history of pelvic infections, ectopic pregnancy or suffer from heavy bleeding, then you should choose some other form of birth control.

Diaphragm or Cap

The diaphragm (sometimes called the Dutch cap) is a disc of rubber that is fitted into the vagina to prevent sperm from reaching the Fallopian tubes. It's inserted before intercourse with lots of contraceptive cream to seal it in. It's a good method of birth control for older women and inexpensive too, since both the cap and cream are available free on the NHS. Diaphragms need to be renewed every year to be completely effective.

Sheaths/Condoms

The male sheath or condom is used externally to cover the penis during intercourse and prevent your partner's sperm from entering your vagina. It's freely available (you can buy condoms over the counter in chemists and many other large stores) and is the best protection against the HIV virus. It's safe to use and has no side effects, but it may be less reliable than some of the other methods described here; if your partner's sheath bursts during intercourse you may need to use emergency contraception (see opposite).

There is now a female sheath (called Femidom) which is becoming more available from family planning centres. It consists of a tube of polyurethane which fits inside the vagina and has a ring at the upper end to keep it in place. As it becomes more widely available, and provided it proves effective, it could become a valuable preventative against AIDS.

Sheaths are probably most convenient if you only need occasional protection. If you don't have a regular partner (or if you have several partners) even if you already use another form of contraception, you might want to consider using a sheath as well, to give you added protection against HIV. (Most other 'barrier' methods of contraception give some protection against HIV but the sheath does offer a more complete protection than the others.)

Vaginal Ring

The vaginal ring (called Fem-Ring) is a progestogen-containing device that is inserted into the vagina on the first day of your period and left there for three months – after this time, you'll need a new one. It can sometimes fall out and you'll need to remember to put it back if it does; otherwise it's reliable and comfortable to wear.

It provides a regular daily dose of progestogen and may sometimes cause irregular bleeding or stop your periods. If you use a vaginal ring, it can sometimes be difficult to know if you are in the menopause – check with your doctor when you're having it replaced if you aren't sure. A vaginal ring will not give you any protection against hot flushes.

Contraceptive Injections

If you don't like taking pills, or are worried that you might forget to take them, or if you can't use the other methods listed above, then injections can provide a safe form of contraception. These are usually given in the buttock and by a doctor or nurse; of the most common injections, Depo-Provera will last about 12 weeks and Noristerat about eight weeks.

Emergency Contraception

This used to be called the 'morning after' pill, although it can be used up to 72 hours *after intercourse*. Obviously this type of birth control should not be used regularly but it can help if you have a problem with your normal method. It works by taking two high-dose contraceptive pills as soon as possible after intercourse, then two more 12 hours after that – the timing is important and you may have to set your alarm clock to keep to the schedule. If you vomit up any of

117

these, you will need to take two further pills. Emergency contraception can also be obtained by inserting an IUD – this works up to five days after intercourse.

Sterilisation

The most extreme – and the most permanent – form of contraception is sterilisation. When you're younger and your need is to postpone your family rather than make sure you never have one, this is not really an option for most people, but as you get older, and if your family is complete, it becomes a more attractive possibility. Nowadays in Britain, it has become one of the most popular forms of contraception for the over 40s age group.

Both men and women can be sterilised. Male sterilisation is called vasectomy and involves cutting the *vas deferens* through which sperm travels to the penis from which it is ejaculated into the vagina. Vasectomy is a minor operation and can be done on a day-care basis. It isn't immediately effective, though, so you should continue taking precautions for a few months afterwards, until all of your partner's stored sperm has gone.

Female sterilisation is more complicated and involves 'tying' the Fallopian tubes in order to prevent fertilisation of the egg. It is not a particularly serious operation these days although you may have to stay in hospital overnight; it's usually done via a laparoscope (see page 159).

Both types of sterilisation are pretty much irreversible, so it is essential that you are absolutely sure about having it done before you embark on it. Being sterilised will *not* bring on the menopause and you will continue to have periods in the usual way.

COPING WITH COMMON GYNAECOLOGICAL PROBLEMS

❝ *I've always been a bit tense when I've had to have a vaginal examination and until recently I'd put off having one if at all possible – it always hurt. But I've been having some problems, so my friend suggested that I went to a well-woman clinic; the nurse there examined me and helped me to relax. She said that the tightness I felt was due to my vaginal muscles being tense. (This is called vaginismus.)*

I'd never even heard of endometriosis until my doctor told me I had it. I'd had pains off and on for a couple of years just before my period and immediately after it started. I was relieved to know what it was and to be taken seriously – part of the time I thought I was imagining it all and the other part I'd convinced myself I had some sort of awful cancer.

When my doctor told me I had thrush I felt so ashamed. It's one of those sexual diseases isn't it. But she was very nice and explained there were other ways to catch it and that it was easily treated. Now I'm just more careful and so far there's been no recurrence. 99

The very things that make us different from men (and in particular our vagina and womb) can cause health problems from time to time, and as our reproductive need for them fades, we should take particular care of them.

Our vagina in particular can be affected by the menopause (see pages 87 to 88) and even if we don't suffer symptoms like vaginal dryness, the muscles that help keep it flexible do weaken with age, which can make us more prone to displacement of various organs around it. And the wall of the vagina becomes less resistant to infection.

If your vaginal muscles have become very weakened and slack (childbirth sometimes starts off

this process which then becomes progressively worse) your doctor may suggest an operation called a colporrhaphy, which involves stitching up and strengthening them. However, very few vaginal problems are as serious as that, and although some can be irritating and uncomfortable, most can be eased or even prevented by exercises and good hygiene.

Vaginal Infections

The best form of cure is prevention, and in the case of vaginal infections, you can help cut down the risks by:

△ using only your own bath towels and wash cloth

△ cleaning the bath and shower after each use

△ rinsing the bath with water if you use chemical cleaners – traces can linger and irritate the delicate vaginal skin, which can lead to infection

△ keeping your vaginal area clean by washing with a little superfatted soap and water regularly – having baths makes this particularly easy

YOUR GENITAL ORGANS

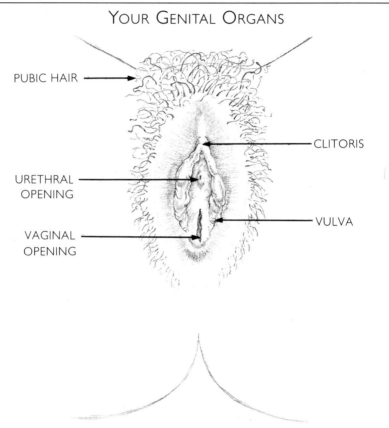

PUBIC HAIR

CLITORIS

URETHRAL OPENING

VAGINAL OPENING

VULVA

Vaginas are usully only about 7.5-IOcm (3-4 inches long) but they enlarge when sexually aroused and vary widely in appearance. Through them eggs are fertilised and babies born (unless you have a caesarian of course), and it is through your vagina that the blood flows each month which helps keep your womb healthy when you are not pregnant.

The opening to your vagina is protected by external folds of skin and fat called the labia (lips). The clitoris, sometimes called a woman's penis (although it's much smaller than that), is a tiny knob of tissue situated under the skin fat just above the opening of the bladder. Like the penis, it becomes swollen with blood during intercourse. You pass urine from your bladder through the urethra, a thin tube closed by a ring of muscle below the bladder. The action of urinating relaxes the muscle and allows the water to pass through.

△ not using bath salts, foam baths or oils, or vaginal deodorants or sprays – they can lead to inflammation of the delicate lining of the vagina, which can be difficult to cure.

The most usual way of transmitting vaginal and urinary infections is sexually. It obviously helps, therefore, to use a barrier method of contraception, to limit the number of your sexual partners and to try to make sure that they are free from infection before you become involved with them.

Antiseptics are sometimes recommended as treatments for vaginal problems but they can make them worse.

The most common vaginal infections are listed below, together with their major symptoms and cures.

THRUSH is probably the most common infection of all and can be transmitted sexually or by using towels or even toilet seats immediately after someone who already has it. The most common symptoms are a genital itch and a white creamy discharge. Thrush responds to pessaries, ointments or tablets and can normally be cleared up quickly once treatment is started. If you would prefer to try a more informal treatment first, an effective home remedy can be live yoghurt applied inside the vagina – the lacto-bacillus in the yoghurt contains a beneficial germ that kills off the thrush bacteria.

VAGINAL TRICHOMONAD also called TV (trichomoniasis vaginalis) is similar to thrush and can be caught in the same way. Its most usual symptom is a smelly discharge. It can be cured by taking Metronidazole tablets twice a day for seven days – avoid alcohol completely (stop the night before you start treatment), when you are taking these tablets since the combination may give you a nasty headache and possibly nausea as well.

GONORRHOEA is almost exclusively a sexual disease and a very common one. For many women there are few symptoms, although sometimes there can be a smelly discharge and, in its acute form, it can be painful to urinate. Gonorrhoea is easily and quickly treated in its early stages (usually with antibiotics) but if it is not treated it can lead to infection of the Fallopian tubes and, in extreme cases, to sterility. Since it is transmitted sexually and is very infectious, if you do have it, you will be asked to name your partner or partners so that they can be tested and treated too.

CHLAMYDIA is similar to gonorrhoea and is treated in the same way.

GENITAL HERPES is another common infection, usually transmitted sexually. It is extremely infectious and if you have reason to believe you have it, you should warn your partner(s) and get treatment as quickly as possible. You will be given tablets (usually to take about five times daily for about five days) or creams – both are effective; although creams to treat herpes are currently only available on prescription, they will soon be available over the counter. If your herpes doesn't clear up when treated as above, you should go back to your doctor or, if you prefer, a genito-urinary clinic to get further treatment.

Resistant herpes can be a sign of infection with the HIV virus.

Vaginal Prolapse

❝ I felt very uncomfortable down below – a pressing feeling – and before I got treatment I'd leak (urine) if I ran or coughed. I had an operation and now it's fine. It was really worth it for me. ❞

Sometimes your vaginal muscles weaken and instead of supporting your womb, bladder and rectum in their normal position in your body, they allow them to bulge into your vaginal cavity. This is called prolapse and the main sign that this might be happening is a general feeling of 'something coming down'. The womb and vaginal wall may descend into the vaginal cavity but cystocele (descent of the bladder) and rectocele (bulging of the rectum) are not uncommon.

All three conditions can be improved by having an operation where a 'tuck' is taken in the vaginal wall and the underlying muscles are strengthened. For prolapse sufferers who don't want to have an operation, a vaginal ring can provide support, although it needs to be replaced every year. If you have to wear a ring, oestrogen cream is useful to strengthen the walls of the vagina and prevent infection.

Bladder and Urethra Problems

The bladder and urethra muscles, like those in the vagina, can also lose some of their strength with age, which can lead to increased vulnerability to infection and to general urinary problems. Like similar problems of the vagina, most of these are easily treated and, with good hygiene and exercise, risks can be minimised.

CYSTITIS Cystitis is a bladder infection, common at any age; it's sometimes called the 'honeymoon disease' because it often occurs after frequent sexual intercourse. Urinating can be painful and so, sometimes, is sex. If you are experiencing pain during intercourse and you have cystitis, it may help to empty your bladder immediately before and after; drinking lots of water can also help. If it's causing recurrent problems, your doctor can prescribe a tablet (Trimethoprim) which can be taken before intercourse to prevent infection. A short course of Trimethoprim is a good treatment for cystitis.

URETHRAL SYNDROME is an infection which is caused by soreness and cracking of the opening of the urethra. It is more common among older, postmenopausal women and signs include painful and frequent urination and a genital itch. HRT in any form prevents urethral syndrome; even if you don't want to take HRT tablets or patches, an HRT cream applied to the offending area should help the problem.

INCONTINENCE can affect women throughout their life, but as you get older and your muscles weaken, it can become more of a problem. *Urge incontinence* is the name given to the condition in which you feel an urge to pass urine suddenly and unpredictably. This can happen through fear or stress – or without any discernible reason. If you feel it happening to you, try to control the flow using pelvic floor exercises (see page 59).

Stress incontinence is the term used to describe a slight, involuntary passing of urine when you cough, sneeze, laugh or exercise. This is an extremely common condition and more embarrassing than anything else; it is caused by a weakening of the sphincter muscle which closes off the outflow of urine from the bladder – and damage to the pelvic muscles while giving birth can lead to this eventually. Pelvic floor exercises can help here too.

If the amount of urine you pass is causing problems, then you should see your doctor who might recommend a small operation to repair the vaginal wall (see page 122).

Other Gynaecological Problems

PREMENSTRUAL SYNDROME is a common complaint in women and is sometimes linked to the swings in hormone levels that occur during the menstrual cycle. What is generally known as PMS or PMT can include headache, depression, bloating, feeling cold and sluggish, weight gain, acne, irritability and aggression; symptoms usually occur for a week or ten days before the period, reaching a peak as you begin to bleed.

Keeping a menstrual chart (see page 81) will help to identify the problem; if you find that your symptoms continue throughout the month then the chances are that you aren't suffering from premenstrual syndrome alone but that your problem is one of chronic anxiety or depression which gets worse in the week before the period.

If you do suffer from premenstrual symptoms there is no instant cure but you can lessen the problem considerably by reducing stress, eating regularly and healthily, and avoiding alcohol during your pre-menstrual week. Occasionally doctors do prescribe drugs similar to aspirin and, if your problem is particularly severe, hormone tablets or antihormones such as Danazol can cure it, although this may change your menstrual cycle. Diuretics can be useful if you suffer from fluid retention.

PMT usually disappears at the menopause. If you've had a hysterectomy where you keep your ovaries you may continue to suffer PMT symptoms since PMT is tied to your ovarian cycle rather than your menstrual one.

ENDOMETRIOSIS is a condition where small pieces of the lining of the womb become embedded in the ovaries, Fallopian tubes, bladder or bowel. It can happen at any time during your fertile life. It's very painful and symptoms can last from the week before your period through the first two days of it. Theoretically it should disappear at the menopause, although it probably won't if you take HRT – HRT can, in

124

fact, sometimes make endometriosis worse.

If you suspect you have it, alert your doctor – it *can* be treated, usually with Danazol if it's considered a fairly minor version; if your pain is very severe, you will probably be sent for a laparoscopy to confirm the extent of the problem. If the condition is serious enough an operation such as hysterectomy is sometimes recommended.

FIBROIDS are lumps of muscle that grow in the wall of the womb – if they're large enough they bulge into the womb cavity itself and the womb increases in size. In some women they produce no symptoms, but they can be a cause of heavy bleeding. If they do, or if they are interfering with your bowel or bladder, a hysterectomy may be recommended.

If you have fibroids but they aren't causing any real problem, it may be better to leave them as they are; after menopause, when you will have less oestrogen to help them grow, they will probably shrink. HRT can make fibroids grow, however, so if you have this problem you need to balance the risks before deciding whether to take it or not.

OVARIAN CYSTS Ovarian cysts are bags of fluid attached to the ovary – they can be any size from a thumbnail to a football. They are usually harmless but they can sometimes be rather a nuisance since they can press on the bladder and bowel. Occasionally a cyst can contain cancerous tissue – so if one is suspected, your doctor may suggest doing some tests such as pelvic ultrasound or laparoscopy (see page 159) to make sure that it does not. If a cyst *is* large, it's usually removed for further examination so that a diagnosis can be confirmed.

Many of us won't have any of the problems spelled out above, and those of us who do will hopefully experience only one or two and these only slightly. But it is nevertheless important for all of us to keep healthy. We are potentially at risk (as we are at any age), and we owe it to ourselves to do what we can to help ourselves stay healthy and vigorous. As always, the key idea can be summed up very simply:

**PREVENTION IS
BETTER THAN CURE!**

125

CHAPTER SIX

HORMONE REPLACEMENT THERAPY – FACTS AND FALLACIES

IS IT A MIRACLE DRUG? *CAN* IT

MAKE US ALL LOOK LIKE JOAN COL-

LINS – OR AT LEAST 20 YEARS

YOUNGER THAN WE ARE? *WILL* WE

BE ABLE TO TAKE IT FOR THE REST

OF OUR LIVES? *DOES* IT STOP HOT

FLUSHES? *CAN* IT STOP US FROM

GETTING OSTEOPOROSIS LATER ON?

One of the most important decisions you will make as you enter the menopause is whether or not you will take HRT (hormone replacement therapy). Although there has been a lot of talk about what it is (and isn't) and what it does (and doesn't), our general level of real information about this treatment is still woefully low; this chapter, therefore, concentrates on presenting the facts as they are known to help you make your choice as informed as possible.

WHAT IS HRT?

HRT is just what it says it is – a treatment which 'replaces' the hormones which, by the time you've reached your menopause, your body is either not producing at all or is producing very much less of.

The hormone that is 'replaced' is oestrogen, whose protective functions are outlined on page 76. As we have also explained, *falling* levels of oestrogen cause some of the common symptoms of menopause, such as flushes and night sweats.

It works very simply: by restoring your supply of oestrogen to the levels you had as a younger, fertile woman, HRT continues the protection against thinning bones and heart disease that a regular high pattern of the hormone gave you in earlier years (see Chapter Four for an explanation of how this protection lessens during and after menopause). And by effectively 'ignoring' the menopause in hormonal terms, it also lessens (and often prevents) immediate menopause symptoms and discomforts such as hot flushes, night sweats and vaginal dryness.

And just as your body manufactures progesterone during your fertile years to protect the lining of your womb, so HRT treatments often include a special short monthly course of synthetic progesterone (progestogen) to continue this during and after the menopause. It's added to prevent the oestrogen in the treatment from over-stimulating the lining of your womb because if this happens, it could lead (comparatively rarely, but it does happen) to cancer of the lining of the womb (endometrial cancer).

HRT comes in many shapes and types and sizes, and what it physically consists of will depend on whether you're talking about a pill, a patch, an implant, a pessary or a cream, and then what

127

type of pill, patch, implant, pessary or cream. Mostly the treatments consist of synthetic oestrogens made in the laboratory (largely because the supply of 'natural' oestrogen couldn't possibly meet the demands of the market) but some are derived from plants such as yams, and there is even one (it's one of the commonly used ones, called Premarin) which is based on the urine of pregnant mares.

There are lots of different ways of taking HRT and both the method of ingestion and the individual dose can differ depending on which type and brand you use. A list of the most commonly used pills, patches, implants, pessaries and creams are given on pages 135 to 145, together with some pros and cons for each method.

WHAT ARE THE BENEFITS?

“ I don't see what the benefits can be. Our mothers got by without any treatment and my mother is very well at eighty.

I quite like the idea of taking it but I do worry about the fact that it, well, interferes with nature somehow. I mean do you have to take it to stay well? ”

The benefits of HRT can be summed up as follows:

△ it helps protect you against thinning bones (osteoporosis)

△ it reduces your risk of heart disease

△ it decreases your chances of having vaginal dryness

△ it lessens hot flushes and night sweats.

HRT is also popularly believed to lessen emotional problems associated with the menopause, but as we have explained on pages 88 to 89, these are more connected with life problems and lifestyle than with biology, and HRT would not necessarily directly affect them.

The most commonly acknowledged benefit of HRT is that it lessens the risk of developing osteoporosis. The protection is immediate – as we have mentioned in Chapter Four, from the time you start to take HRT you stop losing bone density, and if you take it for, say, five years, your bones will be as strong at the end of that time as they were at the beginning.

Since about one woman in four in this country will suffer from a fracture of one sort or another in later life, this is very good news. Some of these fractures can be very serious (fracture of the thigh or hip, for instance) and one, fracture of the spine, is incurable, because the wedged vertebra become deformed and once deformed they can't be straightened even if your bones *do* become thicker again.

The downside is that HRT is effective only while you continue to take it; when you *stop* taking it your bones will begin to thin again, and they will thin at the same rate they did when you reached the menopause.

The other generally agreed benefit to using HRT is that it reduces the risks of heart disease. After the menopause the composition of your blood chemicals gradually change and your blood clots more easily; your blood vessels themselves become tougher and less elastic. Women who have hysterectomies where their ovaries are removed are particularly vulnerable to these changes since, in their case, the change is sudden and abrupt rather than gradual. By taking oestrogen, your cholesterol levels are reduced, your blood vessels will become less rigid and more elastic – and you will be less likely to have a heart attack.

As before, however, HRT is basically most effective while you take it; research suggests that while risks are reduced by about 50 percent while you are on the therapy, protection falls to only about 10 percent after you stop the treatment.

The above protection comes mostly from oestrogen rather than a combination of oestrogen plus progestogen; if you take a combined dose (as most women in this country who have a natural menopause do) then the benefits may not be so great, although the addition of progestogen does not eliminate the protection altogether. Large-scale research is now going on to measure more exactly what difference the addition of progestogen to the therapy makes in this situation so that we will know more definitely what the best options will be.

Since women who have had a hysterectomy take oestrogen-only treatment the above provisos do not apply to them; where their health is concerned, the benefits are clear and acknowledged.

Is it the Elixir of Youth?

❝ Is it like a cosmetic? All these film stars seem to boast about taking it – and they do look wonderful.

Will it get rid of my wrinkles and make me look young again? ❞

There is a popular belief that one of the major benefits of HRT is that it will make you look and feel younger, and give you more energy. Sad to say, this one *does* seem to be myth rather than fact: there is NO evidence to prove that it does.

Research suggests that continued supplies of oestrogen help keep skin moist and flexible, and it is possible that this might affect skin tone, leading to that HRT 'glow' that women's magazines talk about (although many women who don't take HRT but who look after their skin, also 'glow'). Other than that, there is nothing to suggest that it will rejuvenate you, or that it will suddenly give you lots of boundless energy – this state is more likely to happen (when it does) from the relief of discovering that the menopause is here, that it's not so terrible and that you're coping just fine!

WHAT ARE THE DISADVANTAGES?

There are two different types of risk attached to taking HRT, the risk of side effects and the ultimate question of whether the treatment itself is safe – and for how long.

The Side Effects of HRT

❝ The days before the period I feel terrible and very bloated. I usually get a headache and then the period comes – this has been going on for a while now. Aren't there any new treatments that don't cause periods?

Is it supposed to make you put on weight? I've put on over a stone since I started it and I don't seem to be able to get rid of it. ❞

Many people have no problems with HRT at all but others do experience discomfort that can range from minor to major – and in rare cases, serious enough problems to stop the treatment altogether.

Perhaps the most common unwelcome side effect of the combined oestrogen-progestogen HRT package is that you have a monthly period again – not usually a particularly welcome thought when you're over 50 and believed you'd finished with all that! And with the period can come some of the familiar irritating premenstrual-type symptoms and side effects such as bloating, breast swelling and tenderness, nausea, water retention and weight gain.

Most of these problems occur primarily during the initial weeks of treatment and should disappear after the first two or three months. But if you are taking HRT and suffer severely from any of the above – and are still suffering by the end of the first three months – you should go back to your doctor to discuss the situation with him or her. Often symptoms can be minimised or even cured by switching to a different type of treatment, and weight gain and bloating can often be helped by taking diuretics. It's worth investigating further and trying to do something about it if you want to persevere with the therapy.

Is HRT Safe?

66 *I'd like to take it but I'm really scared by all the publicity about it having no safety record – IS it safe?* 99

This, of course, is the $64,000 question. The short answer is that HRT has been used successfully in America for over 50 years and has a generally good safety record. But having said that there are some areas of concern about its use, and there are some potential problems it can raise. You should know about these as you consider whether you want to start taking it or whether you want to continue taking it.

BREAST CANCER Breast cancer is one of the most common cancers in Britain, so anything that increases the risk here is cause for real concern. The current state of research (and there is a great deal of it now going on in this area) suggests that, in the short term HRT definitely *does not* increase the risk of contracting breast cancer. Longer-term British, Swedish and American studies have shown, however, that *prolonged* use can increase your chances of developing this disease, and that the longer you stay on HRT the more the risk increases – the Swedish study showed, for instance, that there was no increased risk up to six years; between six and nine years there was a slight increase; and after nine years, the risk was about one and a half times greater than if you hadn't taken it at all. A similar American study suggested that this last level of risk occurred only after about 20 years of use.

The response by doctors to all of this is generally to offer HRT to all women *at the menopause* who would like it, for an initial period of between five and six years. After this, prescriptions are only renewed if a mammogram is normal (that is, you don't have any signs of breast cancer); see also the box on page 107.

On the whole, many doctors prefer not to prescribe HRT to women who are still menstruating regularly, since they feel that those first precious five or six years of no added risk at all should be used at or after the menopause when it will be most effective and most needed to help protect your bones.

Women who have had their ovaries removed are in a slightly different category. If you've had this type of operation, your chances of developing breast cancer are reduced by 50 percent anyway, so even if you take HRT for many years your chances of contracting the disease will still

be much lower. Many women who have had hysterectomies with removal of ovaries remain on HRT for 20 years or even longer, since the benefits in their case do so clearly outweigh the risks.

OTHER CANCERS When oestrogen-only HRT first began to be prescribed about 20 or 30 years ago, there was some evidence that the treatment increased the risks of developing cancer of the lining of the womb (endometrial cancer). With the addition of progestogen to the HRT package, however, this risk has now disappeared. If you take oestrogen-only HRT (and you haven't had a hysterectomy), you should have a biopsy each year to make sure that it's safe for you to continue with this type of therapy.

CLOTTING PROBLEMS Synthetic oestrogens have been known to increase the risk of thrombosis since studies were first done on the contraceptive pill (which also has synthetic oestrogen as its base). Studies to date on HRT – which is a different type of oestrogen to the one used in the contraceptive pill – have, however, uncovered no evidence to suggest that you run any increased risks of blood clotting while on the treatment. There is some suggestion that because patches don't enter your system via your liver (as pills do) they are extra safe to take, but it is too early to draw conclusions from research done so far.

BLOOD PRESSURE PROBLEMS
Even if you suffer from high blood pressure and take tablets for this, you can still take HRT. However, your doctor or nurse should measure your pressure before you start the treatment, then at intervals for the first year and thereafter once a year, to make sure that levels stay normal. If your blood pressure is high at that first check, you'll probably be given medication or advice to get it back to normal before you begin HRT.

FIBROIDS AND ENDOMETRIOSIS
Fibroids can grow and endometriosis can get worse if you take HRT – so if you suffer from either of these conditions, you'll need to consider carefully before you start treatment. If you do decide to go ahead, make sure that you're monitored closely and stop the therapy if it appears to be making them worse.

What Are the Risks for Me?

" Are there any side effects? My sister has breast cancer and I wouldn't like to run any risks.

I'm still on the pill and my doctor says I should stay on it for a year after my last period. Can I start HRT while I'm still on it?

I smoke two packets of cigarettes a day and my doctor took me off the contraceptive pill when I was 40. I want to take HRT but I'm worried in case I can't take it either. "

For most of us, to take or not to take HRT is a reasonably straightforward personal choice, but some of us are more at risk of developing problems if we take it than others. You are more at risk if you:

△ have already had breast cancer or if you have a family history of breast cancer (that is, your mother or sister have had it)

△ have a severe kidney or liver disease

△ suffer from a deep vein thrombosis or other severe clotting disease, such as lung embolism

△ have fibroids or endometriosis

△ have active gall bladder disease, although it may be possible to use patches in this case

△ are about to have a major operation like a hip replacement where there will be an increased risk of blood clotting.

If you're still taking the contraceptive pill, it's not so much that you shouldn't take HRT as that you don't need it. Contraceptive pills, too, give doses of oestrogen, so you're already getting protection for your bones and help in preventing flushes. HRT can be taken in addition to the contraceptive progestogen only 'mini-pill' if you want some protection against hot flushes and osteoporosis.

For some of the conditions mentioned above, the risks are relatively minor but you should be aware of them as you weigh up the pros and cons of treatment; others are temporary – if you are to have a major operation, for instance, your doctor may be quite happy to have you continue with HRT before you have it (doctors are divided on the advisability of stopping beforehand, although many recommend that you stay off it for a month before you have the operation) – and if you do stop, you can resume the treatment after you've recovered.

TAKING HRT

So you've read all the literature, checked various friends and now you've decided to take the plunge – and the therapy. How do you start?

△ BEFORE you begin, you should visit your doctor to tell him or her of your decision and to discuss any implications it might have. You should make sure that you're given a thorough examination and that your medical history is checked through to make sure that there's no compelling reason why you *shouldn't* take it (see above); many women combine this visit with a general medical check-up and get a breast examination and general physical at the same time (your doctor may suggest this anyway). It's also useful to have had a recent cervical smear and mammogram. See Chapter Five for more specific information on these.

△ DURING initial treatment, you should report back to your doctor after about three months so that both of you can make sure that everything is all right and that you aren't suffering any side effects. This is when minor adjustments may be made to the dose you're taking, or you may switch from one type of treatment to another. After this initial return visit, you should have a check up once a year to make sure that everything continues to be all right.

△ AFTER FIVE OR SIX YEARS both you and your doctor may want to reassess your situation. Normally these days if everything is normal and you remain comfortable taking the prescription, then the recommendation will be to continue taking it (assuming you *want* to continue taking it), with a three-yearly mammogram to make sure that you're free from breast problems. Many American women have been taking HRT for 15 or 20 years or longer with no ill effects and the trend is probably towards more prolonged use here too, if it suits you. If you've had a hysterectomy, the advantages of taking HRT will almost always outweigh the disadvantages, and it's not uncommon to take it for 20 years or more.

WHAT TYPE OF HRT SHALL I TAKE?

The very range of choices can increase your confusion when it comes to choosing what type of treatment to take – there are pills, patches, implants, pessaries and creams to choose from and then different brands of all of these; in the end the choice is a personal one, bearing in mind your own preferences and medical background.

Pills and How They Work

❝ *I'd quite like to take the pills but I'm worried in case I forget to take them – I think I'd find it easier to take one every day rather than stop and start again after a period. Are there any that I could have?*

I feel much better now that I'm on these tablets. It's easier to sleep now that the flushes and sweats are gone – I only get one or two a day.

My breasts feel very sore – could you have a look at them? And could I please try another sort of pill to see if it helps?

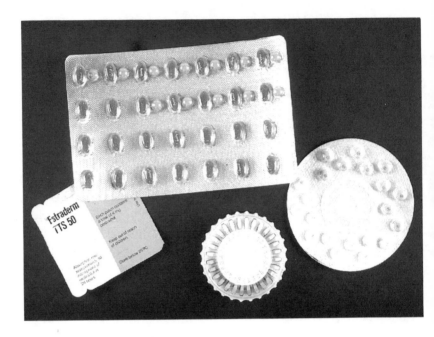

Yes please, could I have another prescription? I feel much better, and deal with my work much better too – I'm a PE teacher. **99**

There are many different HRT pills and patches on the market these days – the above represent a sampling of those available.

The HRT pill is taken orally and usually continuously. Women who have had a natural menopause, take an oestrogen pill every day and, in addition, a progestogen one for about 10–12 days each month – this balances their functions in the same way as their naturally occurring hormones once did (see page 76); after the progestogen course is complete an artificial period occurs. The period isn't a heavy one and usually lasts for roughly five days, after which the treatment cycle starts again.

There is a lot of on-going research to try to find ways of avoiding these monthly 'periods' – and results are cautiously encouraging: in one study, 70 percent of the women who took a course of special combination pills (they were all at least a year

136

COMMON HRT PILLS

FOR WOMEN WHO HAVE HAD A NATURAL MENOPAUSE

▲ Prempak C

0.625mg (red) or 1.25mg (yellow) oestrogen tablets daily plus 12 × 15 microgram brown progestogen (norgestrel) tablets; the norgestrel tablets are taken for the last 12 days of each pack of 28 days. A period usually occurs within three days of stopping the norgestrel. The dose prescribed will vary according to the severity of menopausal symptoms – women who've had more severe ones, and also young women (under 45) who have had the menopause may be given the larger dose.

▲ Cyclo-progynova

11 beige or white oestrogen-only tablets, followed by 10 brown tablets containing oestrogen plus norgestrel. This course comes in two strengths: 1mg oestrogen plus 25 micrograms of norgestrel or 2mg oestrogen plus 50 micrograms of norgestrel. The combinations are taken for 21 days, after which you usually have a period. The larger dose offers full protection to your bones, the smaller one only partial, but the latter is sometimes used for women who have side effects with the larger dose.

CONTINUED OVERLEAF

COMMON HRT PILLS CONTINUED

▲ Trisequens

Strengths range from 0.5–2.00mg (oestrogen) plus 1.00mg progestogen (norethisterone). The course consists of 12 blue oestrogen tablets followed by 10 white oestrogen plus norethisterone tablets then 6 red oestrogen ones and therefore offers a continuous cycle of oestrogen (at different levels) throughout a 28-day monthly cycle. A light bleeding occurs somewhere between about day 23 and day 28.

▲ Nuvelle

2mg white oestrogen-only pills for 16 days then 2mg oestrogen plus 75 micrograms of norgestrel pink ones for 12 days – so this too is a continuous course. Bleeding occurs at the start of each new pack.

▲ Livial

A new preparation, which combines the action of oestrogen, progestogen and testosterone. One 2.5mg white tablet daily. This tablet is supposed to avoid the necessity of having a period although some women have spot bleeding on it, particularly during the early months of use. It does reduce hot flushes, however, and some studies show that it also cuts down the risk of osteoporosis. But it probably doesn't help prevent heart disease.

COMMON HRT PILLS *CONTINUED*

FOR WOMEN WHO HAVE HAD A HYSTERECTOMY

▲ Premarin — Comes in two strengths 0.625mg (red) or 1.25mg (yellow) and is taken daily. Most women take the smaller dose, although those who suffer from particularly severe flushes and those who've had their ovaries removed are often given the larger one. Premarin is the oldest of the pills and nearly all the American studies which have shown the protection offered by long-term HRT have been carried out on patients taking it.

▲ Progynova — Comes in two strengths Img (beige) or 2mg (blue) and is taken daily. The smaller dose doesn't offer full protection against osteoporosis.

▲ Climaval — Comes in two strengths Img (grey) or 2mg (blue) and is taken daily. As with Progynova, the smaller dose doesn't offer full protection against osteoporosis.

beyond the menopause) avoided having periods. Now the hunt is on for the combination that will give 100 percent!

The combination of oestrogen and progestogen is usually the recommended one in the UK. In the United States oestrogen-only pills *are* available for women who have had a natural menopause. These work in the same way as the oestrogen plus progestogen ones except that there is no period at the end of each month. The slight extra cancer risk is dealt with by having a yearly biopsy check to make sure that the womb remains healthy.

Women who have had a surgical menopause and who take the HRT pill, do not need progestogen as part of their treatment since they no longer have a womb. They take oestrogen-only pills every day and don't have a monthly bleed.

Progestogen-only pills are less effective than either oestrogen-only ones, or a combination course, but they can provide some protection against hot flushes and osteoporosis (although they don't help lessen the risk of heart disease), and are therefore sometimes prescribed for people who for one reason or another can't take oestrogen. They are taken daily if you've had a hysterectomy, cyclically otherwise and with a monthly period.

There are many different types of pills: see our tables for the different brands and recommended doses. Milligram doses are given as mg to distinguish them from microgram amounts.

When you go on HRT, your first three monthly bleeds or so may be erratic – this is perfectly normal and is just your body accustoming itself to a monthly menstruation pattern again. After this time your body should have made its adjustments, so if bleeding occurs, especially during the first half of the monthly pill cycle, then you should go and see your doctor.

HRT pills are usually supplied through three-month repeat prescriptions.

Patches – And How They Work

I'd like to try the patches. My friend is on them and she says they're very good except they come off in bed sometimes...

Patches are made from the same type of substances as HRT pills. They are stuck onto the skin (usually the thigh or buttock) twice a week, and are geared to produce a regular daily supply of oestrogen. Because it is absorbed through the skin, a very small dose is effective and in fact it is this method that most closely relates to the way that oestrogen is produced naturally in the body before menopause.

The table on the right summarises the most commonly used HRT patches.

Patches can cause itching or a local rash where they are stuck to the skin, so do try to use a different area each time you use one. Check, too, to make sure that

COMMON HRT PATCHES

FOR WOMEN WHO HAVE HAD A NATURAL MENOPAUSE

▲ Estrapak

Each pack contains eight patches which deliver a daily dose of 50 micrograms of oestrogen, and also 12 1mg red norethisterone tablets – the patches to be fixed to the skin twice a week throughout the cycle and the tablets to be taken during the last 12 days of each pack. Bleeding will usually occur after about 28 days but may come as early as the 26th day – don't worry if it does; the important thing is that the pattern should be regular.

▲ Estracombi

Each pack contains four 50– microgram oestrogen patches and four combined patches (to give a dose of 50 micrograms of oestrogen plus 250 micrograms norethisterone per 24 hours). Apply the four oestrogen packs first, twice weekly, then the combined patches, also twice weekly. Bleeding should occur between days 26–28.

they stay on – they've been known to come off in the shower, or in other places, as you can see from the quote at the beginning of this section! Another way to minimise the chance of itching or rashing is to leave your patch to dry out for 10 seconds before using it – this removes some of the alcohol (used to dissolve the oestrogen) from the mixture and makes the patch sting and itch less when it's put on your skin.

Like HRT pills, bleeding may be erratic at first but everything should have settled down after the first three months. If it hasn't, and doesn't, you should

COMMON HRT PATCHES

FOR WOMEN WHO HAVE HAD A HYSTERECTOMY

▲ Estraderm

This is an oestrogen-only pack and comes in three strengths which deliver a 100 microgram, 50 microgram or 25 microgram dose daily – the middle one is the most usual dose and is known to help prevent osteoporosis; the smallest dose is only partly protective but is often used when there have been troublesome side-effects (breast swelling for instance) with a larger dose. The most usual people to receive the 100 microgram dose are younger women whose ovaries have been removed, or women who are being weaned off an implant – in fact, you may need two 100–microgram patches at once, replaced twice weekly, in order to give you a sufficiently high dose of oestrogen while this is happening initially; the dose is then gradually reduced as your body readjusts. Each pack contains eight patches, which should be fixed onto the skin twice a week.

go to see your doctor. She will probably want to see you after your first three months of treatment anyway, to check on your progress and to find out if there have been any problems. Like pills, HRT patches are usually offered on three-month prescriptions.

Implants and How They Work

Women who have had their womb and ovaries removed have a further choice of how they take HRT: implantation. A hormone pellet – sometimes oestrogen on its own, sometimes with testosterone added – is inserted (usually by your gynaecologist) into the fatty tissue of the wall of the stomach under local anaesthetic. It sounds more dramatic and painful than it is! Each implant is supposed to last for six months then be replaced by a new one, but occasionally one is effective for less time than this so if you've had an implant and feel flushes, sweats or other menopause symptoms coming on, it might be a good idea to have your hormone levels checked.

Implants are known to be very effective in reducing the impact of surgical menopause (hysterectomy) on your body: they help to lessen the sexual problems some women experience at this time, and they also cut down the risk of developing osteoporosis.

Pessaries and How They Work

Pessaries look like small white bullets and, if used to give full protection, should be used daily or twice weekly, depending on the brand. They are mostly made from oestrogen only plus wax or some other harmless material, and because of this they are often recommended for women who have had a hysterectomy. (The vagina absorbs drugs well and oestrogen applied there could over-stimulate the womb for those women who have had a natural menopause.)

Pessaries are probably most valuable when they are used 'locally' that is to treat vaginal problems after the menopause – they are particularly useful in treating vaginal dryness and infection, and they are much less messy to use if you have one of these problems than oestrogen creams.

Oestrogen Creams and How They Work

Creams are usually made from oestrogen mixed with a cream base to give a soft consistency. They are not recommended as a complete HRT treatment and can be quite messy to use – although some women who have problems coping with an artificial period can benefit from them. They are inserted either with an applicator according to package instructions or, if only a tiny dose is required, by the tip of the finger to the vaginal opening.

❝ I don't take HRT and don't want to really but my doctor has suggested that I take an HRT cream because I'm having problems with intercourse. Is this necessary and will there be any problems? ❞

COMMON HRT PESSARIES AND CREAMS

FOR WOMEN WHO HAVE HAD A HYSTERECTOMY

▲ Vagifem — A pessary that gives a dose of 25 micrograms per day. Bought in packs of 15, with doses every day for the first two weeks then twice weekly for the rest of the monthly cycle or as required.

FOR ALL WOMEN

▲ Ovestin

▲ Premarin } All creams should be applied locally

▲ Dienoestrol

Creams are used primarily to treat 'local' problems and are particularly helpful for women who have sexual problems caused by vaginal dryness. If you want to use it to help this particular problem, dab it on to your vaginal opening at a regular time each day (*not* before you have sex; you shouldn't use it just before intercourse – unless of course you want your partner to take HRT as well!). And no, you shouldn't have any problems with it. Have a break every two months to assess whether or not you need it.

Pills versus Patches

The real choice for most women who want to have the full benefit of HRT is whether to use pills or patches – implants aren't used so often these days. Each has its advocates, and each has its advantages and disadvantages. The table on the right will give you an at-a-glance idea of the pros and cons to consider as you make your choice; and of course once you have made the initial decision to take pills or patches, your doctor will be happy to talk it all over with you and

144

ADVANTAGES

PILLS

Proved to reduce risk of osteoporosis

Proved to reduce risk of heart attacks

Prevent flushes (in most women)

Cheap to use

Prevent or lessen vaginal problems

Good (and long) safety record of over 50 years

Period bleeding is controlled

PATCHES

Reduce risk of osteoporosis

Reduce risk of flushes (for most women)

Prevent or lessen vaginal problems

Tiny dose is effective

Do not affect liver proteins and therefore do not affect blood pressure

Are useful if you have digestive problems

DISADVANTAGES

PILLS

May cause indigestion and gall bladder problems

Affect liver proteins and may occasionally raise blood pressure

PATCHES

Possible skin reactions such as rash and itch

Expensive

Sometimes fall off

Bleeding patterns are not so predictable.

recommend the specific varieties within each type most suitable for you.

Patches are much younger than pills – they were introduced during the 80s – and this is the reason we have not marked them as proven to reduce risks of osteoporosis and heart attack (most of the long-term studies have been done on pills, and on Premarin users in particular).

This is not to say that patches are unsafe or that they are any less safe than pills; only that there is, for the moment, much less research evidence on their safety so far.

145

STOPPING HRT

6 6 *I've been on HRT for a couple of years now and I don't particularly want to take it for much longer. But I'm a bit worried about coming off – will I get all the menopause symptoms again when I finally do?*

My doctor has told me that I should come off HRT now because I've been on it for nearly eight years – but I've got a really stressful job and I'm concerned about the side effects when I do. Is there any way to do it gradually? 9 9

At some point, you will probably want to come off HRT for one reason or another. When this time comes, try if at all possible to come off slowly rather than abruptly – halve, then quarter whatever dose you're taking (ie if you're taking oestrogen tablets, take them on alternate days rather than every day, keeping the progestogen course the same, over a period of about three months or so).

When you come off, you'll suffer from flushes, regardless of your age and how long you've taken HRT – coming off slowly, as described above, will make them less severe. The recurrence of flushes doesn't mean you

should go back on oestrogen 'for ever'; they are a withdrawal symptom, are harmless and will eventually disappear.

Try to avoid coming off HRT if you're setting off for a sunshine holiday abroad somewhere – the heat will aggravate the flushes. And if you do have a particularly difficult time looming ahead either in the family or at work, it might be sensible to wait until it's over before you begin your wind-down.

Currently about 9 percent of British women take HRT but this figure is rising – more women are trying it, at least for a while.

Ultimately, though, the decision is a personal one for you to make about yourself, and if you feel that you *don't* want to take this treatment, or if you can't take it for some medical reason, you shouldn't allow your- self to be stampeded into starting against your will or feel that you must consign yourself to a less healthy, frailer future. Although we have shown that HRT does have proven benefits, it is as well to remember that there *are* other ways to protect your bones against thinning and your heart against attack – as the earlier chapters of this book make clear. A healthy diet, moderate exercise and a positive and happy lifestyle can probably do you as much good as any drug can most of the time!

Equally, if you do decide that HRT is for you, then hopefully we have been able to reassure you that HRT *is* safe for most people most of the time, and that providing you look after yourself while you continue taking it, you should be able to enjoy the benefits that it can bring.

Don't feel bad about taking it or not taking it. Talk to friends, doctors and partners and avoid being pressured into anybody else's choice. The decision is yours. Make it a positive one – for you.

CHAPTER SEVEN

HELPING YOU TO HELP YOURSELF

MAINTAINING GOOD HEALTH AND
WELL-BEING, AS YOU'LL ALREADY
HAVE GATHERED, REQUIRES A BIT
OF EFFORT — BUT SINCE YOU WILL
BE THE MAIN BENEFICIARY OF ANY
IMPROVEMENT THAT TAKES PLACE,
IT'S AN EFFORT WELL WORTH
MAKING.

The same is true for those times when you need to get help from others in order to keep yourself healthy – there are ways and there are better ways to deal with our health services! In the pages that follow, we explain how to make sure that you get the best results possible from the 'system,' both public and private, and in a series of questions-and-answers, we try to answer the questions you raise most often about your health and the menopause.

KEEPING HEALTHY

By now, we hope that you will be eating healthily and exercising moderately as a matter of course. But there are also certain other basics for good health which you should be checking on regularly and looking after constantly – like your teeth, your sight and your hearing; you need all three in good working order to enjoy life to the full at any age.

TEETH These are, of course, important for your digestion but they are also a precious asset to your looks and your comfort. Many of us in the past lost our teeth because we didn't bother to look after them, feeling that it

was somehow 'inevitable' that we lost them early on in our adulthood. Don't let this happen to you! Yearly dental checks are good value for money, so make sure that you have one.

Having a baby and also breast feeding drain calcium from your body which can weaken your teeth, so following our recommendations (see pages 62 to 65) for drinking milk and eating calcium-rich foods will not only help you preserve your bones better – it will help you strengthen your teeth as well.

If you've already lost your teeth, make sure that your dentures fit properly and that you keep them in good condition.

Healthy Teeth Tip: Fluoride toothpaste prevents tooth decay and chewing raw fruit and vegetables protects your gums.

EYES Our eyes can let us down a bit as we get older and most people, men and women, find that by their mid-40s their sight has altered and that their eyes focus farther away. The practical result of this is that many of us have to invest in reading glasses or at the very least hold small-print books a long way away from our eyes in order to read them properly. If you find that you're having problems reading – and even if you're not – you should have regular check-ups on your eyes too. A good optician will test you not only for long or short sight but will also check the general health of your eyes.

Healthy Eyes Tip: Make sure that the lights in your home function properly and that there's a good mixture of 'spot' lighting for reading and overhead or wall lights for general illumination. A weak light that's near to you is as good as a stronger one far away. An Anglepoise light that you can adjust to your needs is a good investment.

EARS Deafness can happen at any age and from many causes – infection, catarrh or wax build-up to name a few. Don't attempt home remedies for wax problems; using cotton tips, for instance, can be dangerous. Have a medical check if you're finding it hard to catch what people say, and don't be afraid of using a hearing aid if

you need one; there are lots of very discreet designs you can wear these days, and they are an enormous help in allowing you to participate fully in social or business situations.

Healthy Ears Tip: Wax has a nasty habit of building up in your ears; if you feel deaf, go to your GP's surgery – there will usually be someone there who can help remove more impacted wax. You'll be surprised at the difference a regular clean out can make to your hearing!

CHECKING UP ON YOURSELF
One of the cornerstones of good preventive medicine is an annual check-up, and more and more people are taking advantage of schemes that allow them to have one either privately or through work, or from the increasing number of general practices that now offer a range of well-woman and other preventive clinics.

To be useful, a good check-up should be a mixture of interview, where you'll be asked questions like the ones listed in the box opposite, and examination (see box overleaf).

WHAT HAPPENS AT AN ANNUAL CHECK-UP

THE TYPE OF QUESTIONS YOU'LL BE ASKED

▲ What medication(s) are you taking and how long have you been taking it (them).

▲ The date of your last period, and whether it was regular and/or heavy; and whether you've been 'spotting'.

▲ Whether you've had an operation to remove your womb and ovaries.

▲ Your method of contraception (if applicable).

▲ What your appetite is like and your general ability to work and exercise.

▲ How you feel in yourself; are you under stress?

▲ How much do you drink per week.

▲ Do you smoke? And if you do, how many a day.

▲ Do you get enough calcium in your diet (see pages 62 to 65 to work out your calcium intake).

▲ Do you exercise regularly.

▲ Have you had any major life changes recently, for instance bereavement.

▲ Is there any family history of heart disease, breast cancer, etc.

▲ Do you pass urine too frequently. Can you hold it in?

▲ Do you move your bowels regularly.

THE TESTS/EXAMINATIONS YOU'LL BE GIVEN

▲ Your height and weight will be measured – and you'll be asked if your weight has changed recently.

▲ Your blood pressure will be taken, and your heart rate and rhythm measured.

▲ Your urine will be tested (to see whether it contains sugar, protein or bacteria).

▲ Your cholesterol level will be measured.

▲ A blood test may be taken to check that you aren't anaemic and that your cell count is normal.

THREE-YEARLY EXAMINATIONS YOU SHOULD HAVE

▲ Mammogram (see pages 106 to 109)

▲ Cervical smear test (see page 109)

Many of the questions and the yearly tests will be handled by nurses or other health professionals rather than by doctors, and the atmosphere will be informal and relaxed. Depending on the number of tests you're having, it shouldn't take all that long – certainly no more than a couple of hours.

Your check-up will be even more useful if you prepare for it in advance by working out answers to the questions listed in the boxes (keeping a menstrual chart, for instance, if your period has been irregular).

Often other tests (for thyroid activity or arthritis, or bone density, among others) will be suggested and arranged after this visit – so don't worry if this happens to you. It means that your health practitioners are doing their job and being thorough, not that you necessarily have some dreaded illness!

USING ALTERNATIVE THERAPIES

❝ I don't particularly like the idea of taking pills and other chemical things for my aches and pains – I would rather try and cure them naturally. Would an alternative therapy help?

My friend claimed acupuncture cured her fear of flying – is it any good for anything else? ❞

Many people combine conventional medicine with what are called alternative therapies for specific ailments, or for particular preventive treatment – back pain can often be lessened or cured with the help of a good osteopath, for instance, or stress or premenstrual tension relieved by an aromatherapy massage, and we've all heard of stubborn smokers giving up the weed after a few encounters with an acupuncture needle!

If you feel you would like to try an alternative medicine, make sure that you find a well qualified practitioner (see the national organisations listed on page 179 which will provide a vetted list), and monitor your progress to make sure that your treatment is effective and professionally carried out. You will be asked many of the questions listed here if you consult a complementary health practitioner – and others as well, depending on your reason for consulting him or her – so you'll increase the usefulness of this type of visit, too, if you work out the answers, or assemble your list of symptoms, in advance.

Many GPs are now willing to recommend particular types of alternative medicine for some ailments, and some even work with specific practitioners – for instance osteopaths (for back and other muscle pains), and acupuncturists (for arthritis and addictions, such as smoking). So if you don't like the idea of approaching someone you don't know anything about, but would like to try the therapy, it would be worth checking with your practice to see if it's willing to recommend anyone.

Homoeopathy is another alternative medicine that has many adherents – both the Queen and the Prince of Wales use this treatment. Homoeopathy works on the holistic principle, that is, it treats the whole body rather than just the localised problem that you are seeking help for. Like the other complementary medicines discussed above, the quality of the homoeopath you consult is crucial, so check with the national organisation listed on page 179 to get its list of vetted practitioners if you want to try this therapy.

GOING TO SEE YOUR GP

❝ I really dread going to my GP; I feel nervous and rushed when I'm there because I know there are all these people waiting to see her, and I always assume they're more ill than I am. What can I do to make the most of the time I have with her? ❞

Throughout this book we've stressed that if you're having problems of any sort, or even if you *think* there's something wrong, you should go to see your doctor. But since your time with him or her will be limited, and since he or she isn't a mind reader (although some doctors try hard to be!), you should 'prepare' for your meeting so that you can get the best from it. Try a combination of the following:

△ Write down when your problem started, when it's at its worst and if it's getting worse – and how fast.

△ Write down a list of specific symptoms, including how long they last and in what order they appear or have appeared.

△ Include any physical changes you've experienced recently, whether you think they're relevant or not.

△ If you have a menstrual problem or if you want to check on whether you're entering the menopause or not, keep a menstrual chart for a month or two before you go.

△ Make a note of any medications you're taking or have taken recently, prescription and non-prescription.

△ Make a list of the questions *you* want to ask your doctor during your appointment.

△ Make a note of what *you* think is the cause of your problem, and what you expect him or her to do about it.

Your doctor may want to give you an internal examination (depending on the problem, of course). You don't need to bathe immediately beforehand if you think you're going to have one, nor do you need to powder yourself – talcum powder is a nuisance, in fact, particularly if you're having a cervical smear. Just maintain generally good standards of cleanliness and that will be enough. It may be helpful to carry a fresh tampon or sanitary towel in your bag since the smear test may cause a slight bleed, although most practices will provide you with one if you need it.

Don't be surprised if you don't immediately get a prescription to alleviate your problem. The best doctors will take time to make a diagnosis and may arrange further tests; and they may eventually give you advice or suggest counselling rather than give you a conventional prescription. Accurate diagnosis is important at any time but it's particularly relevant around the time of the menopause when social or psychological problems, or an illness such as anaemia, can overlie the picture of menopausal symptoms and confuse the issue.

If, after talking to you and examining you, your doctor recommends specific treatment, make sure that you understand exactly what it is you'll be doing

or taking and for what. You should know, for instance:

△ what it's for

△ why you're taking it

△ what side effects there might be

△ how long you should take it

△ whether it fits in with any other medicines you're taking

△ whether you should avoid alcohol or certain foods while you're on the treatment

△ how and when you take it – for instance, by mouth or rubbed on skin, before or after meals, last thing at night, and so on.

These aren't idle questions – many women gain weight if they take antidepressants or progestogens, for instance; alcohol can be dangerous if you drink it while you're on a course of antihistamines or antidepressants; and you need to avoid some types of food if you're taking some antidepressants. So ask – and learn! Your doctor is there to help with information, advice and support as well as give out prescriptions.

Communication is a two-way street. Just as it's vital that you understand what your doctor is saying to you, it's equally important that he or she knows what's happening to you. So be honest about how much or how little your symptoms bother you; many unnecessary operations are carried out because people haven't been able to explain properly the extent to which they are experiencing pain.

If you go to your doctor for HRT and he or she refuses to discuss it or consider prescribing it for you (and there's no good medical reason why you can't take it), you can ask to be referred to a consultant who would be willing to give it to you. Some parts of the country have self-referral menopause clinics that you can attend without a letter from your general practitioner and at these, too, you will be able to find out more about the therapy and get a prescription if you want to have one. Your local health authority or local hospital would be able to tell you if there's one in your area, and how to get in touch with it.

If the opposite happens, and you are reluctant while your doctor is overly anxious to get

you on it: *stand your ground and say no*. It's *your* body and if you don't want to take it (and there's no compelling medical reason why you should – see pages 128 to 129), then don't.

VISITING A CONSULTANT OR HOSPITAL DOCTOR

Occasionally your doctor will refer you to a consultant for a second opinion, often a gynaecologist, that is a doctor who specialises in what's generally called women's diseases. It will be a gynaecologist who will perform a D&C or biopsy, for instance, if your general practitioner wants to check whether you have womb problems.

The suggestions given above for preparing for your visit to your GP hold good for an appointment with a consultant; you'll get a lot more out of it if you put more into it.

If you visit a consultant who works with the National Health Service there may be a considerable wait before you can see him or her – another good reason for not waiting too long before going to see your own GP if you have a problem. Most consultants work with specific hospitals, and if you do have a problem they want to check out for you, or if they recommend surgery, then it is very likely that you will be asked to go into this hospital and that the consultant will perform the procedure or operation there.

GOING INTO HOSPITAL

&& I'm 47 and my sex drive has practically disappeared since the operation two years ago. Before it we had a very good sex life and I thought I might get pregnant. I went to see the gynaecologist and asked for a sterilisation. They did this under a general anaesthetic and when I woke up they'd removed the womb, ovaries, everything. I had said that I didn't want a hysterectomy but they're terribly busy and I expect they forgot.

Everybody told me that the D&C was really minor, that I'd feel fine after it. So I didn't bother having someone collect me from the clinic and I arranged lots of meetings at work for the next day. Well, I felt terrible and really weak – I don't know how I managed to get home on my own. As for work – I had to have a couple of days off. I was really annoyed that they'd misled me like that. &&

Going into hospital, however briefly, can be quite traumatic and it doesn't help if you feel that you're not being told about

what will happen to you, or that you're being misled about the seriousness of what will be done. Hospital staff do now make great efforts to keep their patients informed about the technicalities of procedures they'll be undergoing but it is important that you ask questions, and that you keep asking them, until you understand what they're telling you. If possible try to get hold of leaflets or other written information about your operation before you have it so that you can go through them at your leisure.

If you're having an operation of any kind now, you'll be asked to sign what's called a consent form – this is a piece of paper that enables the surgeon to extend the scope of your operation if what he finds when he is performing it, warrants this. In the first case mentioned above, when the surgeon began the sterilisation procedure, he found small cysts on the woman's ovaries; since ovarian cysts can be one of the first signs of ovarian cancer (see page 110), he removed her ovaries and womb to ensure her safety. His actions were perfectly proper in the circumstances, but perhaps a lot of heartache and distress could have been avoided if the possibility of this happening had been clearly explained to his patient (and she had clearly understood the risks) before the operation.

Before *you* sign a consent form in hospital, make sure you know about and completely understand the following:

△ what is being done. Is it a test to confirm a diagnosis? Will anything be removed?

△ *why* it's being done. Is it to remove a lump, to stop pain or bleeding, or to control fertility? Is there another form of treatment that would suit you better?

△ who will carry out the operation

△ how long you will need to stay in hospital

△ how long it will be before you can return to work. Will you need special care at home while you convalesce?

Your doctor, and the hospital, will tell you in advance what you'll need to bring with you if your stay is to be more than an overnight one; and if you require any kind of special diet, kosher, vegan, or wheat-free, for instance, you should warn the hospital in advance of this – when you've recovered a bit from the operation, you'll look forward to mealtimes as a respite from the rather monotonous routine of life in the ward.

The more you know about yourself and your health *before* you start to tackle the health system, the better you'll find your way around it. We've listed below some of the questions that we've been asked most often – and we've tried to give you the fullest answers possible.

Q *My doctor says that I've got to have a biopsy – is this the same as a D&C? My friend had one of these last year.*

A An endometrial biopsy is almost the same as a D&C. Your doctor will recommend a biopsy to check whether you have abnormal endometrial cells or even endometrial cancer. It's usually an outpatient procedure although occasionally overnight admission and a general anaesthetic are arranged. What happens is that a small sample of the womb tissue is obtained by inserting a tiny rotating brush or fine nozzle attached to a syringe; it isn't as terrible as this sounds – it's quite similar to inserting an IUD (coil), in fact. The sample cells obtained in this way are then sent to a laboratory for further examination under a microscope so that an accurate diagnosis can be made.

A D&C (the short name for a procedure called dilatation and curettage) is usually performed under a general anaesthetic, and generally requires an overnight stay. In this case the passage to the cervix is opened up and a small spoon is inserted to scrape away most of the lining of the womb. Your doctor will often suggest a D&C if you suffer from heavy bleeding but, like biopsy, it is basically an exploratory procedure, designed to give the doctor further information to help diagnosis, rather than a cure in itself.

Neither of these operations will leave a scar, and they are minor procedures; you should be home by the day after they're performed at the very latest, and back at work a few days after that.

Q *I want to be sterilised and my doctor has said that he'll use a laparoscope to do it. He did try to explain what it was to me but it didn't make much sense at the time – can you tell me what it is, please?*

A A laparoscope is like a narrow telescope and is inserted into you (through a small cut made below the navel) to enable your doctor to 'see' inside your pelvic area. It's now widely used both to check out any womb or ovary problems and also to tie the Fallopian tubes (female sterilisation). It's a very safe, minor procedure, which can be carried out under a local anaesthetic, although more often a general anaesthetic is given plus an overnight stay.

Q *I'm about to have a hysterectomy and the doctor says I'll be off work for three months and won't be able to 'do' things. Does this include sex? And will it be painful to start again after the operation?*

A The length of time it will take you to recouperate from a hysterectomy will depend to some extent on you and your general health, but three months is about the average you should allow. You won't be totally incapacitated for all of it and as time goes on you'll gradually get stronger and more able to do things. About six or eight weeks afterwards, for instance, you should be able to drive comfortably again and get out and about – although you should try not to carry heavy objects around. For instance, even after you have recovered, don't carry your shopping in one heavy bag; divide the weight between two and carry one in each hand to balance yourself.

As regards sex, there's no reason why you can't resume it about six to eight weeks after the operation, providing you're free of pain and not bleeding. It won't be painful, although both you and your partner will probably be a bit tentative in your efforts not to interfere with your still tender tummy! Don't worry about this; just take it slowly, and gradually you'll realise that it's quite safe and not going to give you any kind of relapse or rupture. If you're a little dry when you start again, use a lubricant to make penetration easier; you can buy them over the counter at any chemist's shop.

Q *I find that I need to go to the toilet more often now than I used to. Is this normal?*

A Bladder control can become less efficient as we get older and urinary frequency means that you need to rush to the toilet more often. If you find that you pass a little urine when you laugh or exercise, this is called stress incontinence (see page 123); the main reason for stress incontinence is weakened pelvic floor muscles caused by childbirth, being overweight or by chronic constipation. Pelvic floor exercises (or Kegel exercises as they're sometimes called) can be used to strengthen these muscles (see page 59).

All of these problems have more to do with general wear and tear than the menopause. However, oestrogen creams can be used to thicken the walls of the urethra and vagina and so help them to resist infection. If symptoms persist, or you are very troubled by them, go and see your doctor who may suggest pessaries if the problem is a minor one, or possibly a surgical repair operation if prolapse of the womb is the cause (see page 122).

Q *I've put on three-quarters of a stone in the last two months. What can I do?*

A Start by looking carefully at what you eat and how much exercise you take – an increase in weight can result from quite a small change in routine. Obviously try to eat a healthy diet (see pages 62 and 63). If you are eating reasonably well generally, then the answer might be to cut out one thing, for instance, the snack you have before you go to bed. It's best to combine a change of diet with some extra exercise to keep in shape as you lose weight.

Weight gain may be due to water retention, especially if your hormones are fluctuating during the menopause. If you think this may be the reason you're putting on weight, cut down on salt and eat foods that are natural diuretics – celery, parsley or grapes are good examples.

If you binge eat or find that you are frequently eating for 'comfort', you may need help to break out of this pattern – the organisations listed on pages 180 and 184 can give you further information and counselling help on this.

Q *I always feel tired in the morning and don't think I get enough sleep – I usually have about five hours. Is this possible?*

A Most adults need about six hours sleep a night, although many (Napoleon and Lady Thatcher among them) seem to manage with much less; we do need less sleep with age, so you shouldn't necessarily worry about having less sleep than you used to. Studies show that we aren't very accurate at estimating how long it takes us to get off to sleep anyway!

If you feel tired all the time you should look at your sleep *pattern* rather than the amount of time you spend asleep. The first stage of sleep lasts about 10 minutes when we doze, half-awake, and dream a little. This merges into a deep sleep which becomes even deeper. After about three hours this becomes REM (rapid eye movement) sleep when we dream and our eyes move rapidly under closed lids. We often have very vivid dreams towards the end of this type of sleep. Both alcohol and sleeping tablets disturb REM sleep and if you take one or both of these, this could explain your daytime drowsiness. Other possible causes for sleeplessness are:

△ *Onset insomnia* – You can't sleep when you go to bed. This can often be due to eating late or excitement, worry or drugs like caffeine in strong tea or coffee.

△ *Early morning waking* – This may be due to depression; you go to sleep but wake up about three o'clock in the morning feeling terrible, and you can't get back to sleep. If this persists you should go to the doctor and get some help.

△ *Cigarettes* – Cigarettes can cause insomnia by interfering with the sleep centres in the brain. The cure for this one is to stop smoking (see page 55)!

△ *Sleeping pills* – No one disputes that sleeping tablets are occasionally useful, but the body gets used to them very quickly and after it does, you can become addicted and they can prevent you from sleeping rather than helping you to sleep. Never take them regularly – use only for emergency situations, such as jet-lag or some similarly important event.

△ *Night flushes and sweats* – Menopausal sweats and flushes often seem worse at night and can interrupt sleep. See page 86 for how to help beat them.

There are some easy ways to combat the above problems, apart from avoiding things like cigarettes, coffee with caffeine and sleeping pills. For instance:

△ Exercise during the day or have an early evening walk – this will relax your muscles and make it easier to drift off to sleep.

△ Take a warm drink before going to bed (avoiding stimulants like caffeine of course); try a herbal tea such as camomile or a milky drink like cocoa or hot chocolate.

△ If you're preoccupied by problems, try to find ways of tackling them during the day.

△ Relax in bed (see the box on page 165). Music, reading and sex can help too.

△ Don't take naps during the day however tired you feel. Relax for 20 minutes instead (see pages 164 to 166).

△ Don't go to bed too early.

△ Don't panic. You'll get enough sleep in the end. Get up, make a drink and read for a while if you really can't sleep.

△ If night sweats are the cause of your sleeplessness, learn a routine to deal with the disruption automatically.

Keeping in mind the following might help:

> **WAKE UP – COOL DOWN – GO BACK TO BED – RELAX – AND REST**

Q *I'm in my early-mid 40s and have recently started suffering from PMT for the first time in my life. Is this to do with the menopause, and is there anything you can suggest that will help?*

A Premenstrual tension, or premenstrual syndrome, the terms used to describe a group of symptoms such as bloated stomach, tiredness, irritability, breast tenderness, tension and sometimes depression, can often affect women in their 30s and 40s. But there may be different types of PMT, and there may be other causes of tension too, such as marital problems, stress or feeling angry, so don't just assume that it *must* be PMT.

It can help to keep a menstrual diary such as the one suggested on page 81. Record your symptoms daily across a couple of cycles so that you can see if there's a definite pattern. Some women have on-going problems that become harder to deal with before a period; others notice more dramatic changes. Usually it's a bit of both, an interaction between your own personal problems and that time of the month.

As yet, there's no clear understanding of the biological causes of PMT. Medical and hormonal treatments work by over-riding or cancelling out the menstrual cycle, but your doctor might prescribe diuretics if bloating is a particular problem (see page 161). Progestogen is a popular treatment, although it has been found to be no better than a dummy pill (placebo) in recent research studies.

If you prefer self-help approaches you could try the following, while monitoring your monthly cycle:

△ practise relaxation, especially before your period

△ take regular exercise – it really can help

△ don't expect to feel bad every month

△ arrange more demanding activities for the good weeks when you can.

Many women say that oil of evening primrose reduces feelings of tension and other PMT symptoms such as breast tenderness; one or two 500mg capsules two or three times a day are usually recommended, but higher doses are safe. Others swear by vitamin B6 (pyridoxine) which is found in whole grains, bran, milk and egg yolk. A balanced diet is important, as is regular food intake, although dietary remedies are as yet being used on a trial basis.

It makes sense if you try any of the above measures, to do them one at a time so that you can tell if they work.

Q *I get a lot of hot flushes and they seem to get worse when I'm tense. How can I learn to relax?*

A Many hot flushes *can* be brought on or made worse by stress or general tenseness but there are other causes too, so the first thing you should do is find out what *does* act as your trigger. You could do this by keeping a diary of your flushes to find out when yours occur and what precipitates them (you could adapt the chart on page 81 for this). In a detailed study of hot flushes in 20 women about half seemed to be triggered by what was going on in their lives. If you can identify your triggers you might be able to take some positive action to reduce the flushes.

Recent studies do suggest that being under stress seems to lower our thresholds for having hot flushes, and flushes increase at times when other problems arise. One woman found that hers became worse after her brother died and, as her grief resolved, her flushes lessened too.

Relaxing will help. Practise daily if you can until you can calm your breathing and relax your muscles fairly easily in a short space of time (see page

164

HOW TO RELAX

Find a comfortable armchair and set aside 20 minutes of undisturbed time. Wear loose clothing and no shoes. Tensing, then loosening, your muscles will help them to relax, and slow, gentle, even breathing will calm your thoughts.

▲ Now close your eyes and take a few deep breaths – from your stomach.

▲ Concentrate on the muscles in your body. Feel yourself resting heavily in the chair as if it would be an effort to move.

▲ Start by tensing your arms and hands tightly for a few seconds – then relax for longer. Let them rest loosely on the chair and imagine the feelings of relaxation flowing down to your fingertips.

▲ Tense your shoulders and back by lifting your shoulders up and back while taking a deep breath. Hold it. And then relax. Let your shoulders rest down as far as they can and your back sink heavily into the chair. Feel the relaxation spreading.

▲ Let your breathing be gentle, passive and even, from your stomach. It should be effortless, just like it is before you drift off to sleep. Each time you breathe out, feel yourself becoming heavier and more relaxed with each breath.

▲ Tense and relax your stomach (by making it tight) and your legs and feet (by stretching them out). Then breathe and relax further.

▲ Rest for a while just following your breathing in an effortless, calm state.

165). There are lots of different ways of achieving relaxation: you have to find one that suits you best. One method is given in the box on page 165, but yoga, meditation or self-hypnosis are all beneficial. It's important to relax your mind as well as your body.

Using your imagination can help you relax too. You could conjure up a calming scene or picture in your mind at the end of the relaxation exercises, for instance, or instead of them. This can help if you're finding it hard to cut off from daily thoughts. For example, by thinking about lying on a beach, floating on still water or watching a river, you can absorb all your senses if you have a good imagination: feel the heat, hear the sounds of the water lapping, see the clouds drift.

Once you've learned the skills of relaxing, you can try to reduce the impact of your flushes by relaxing just as soon as you feel one coming on. Daily practice might well make them less frequent. The way you react to the flushes can make quite a difference as well:

△ keep calm

△ don't panic

△ breathe slowly and deeply

△ remember that they don't last very long

△ remember that you notice them much more than other people do

△ there's nothing whatever to be ashamed of!

Q *I'm absolutely terrified of having a hot flush when I'm in company. What should I do if I'm unlucky enough to have one?*

A Hot flushes can be unnerving if they occur when you're in the middle of a conversation or social occasion. The embarrassment is often because of the fear that the other person might misinterpret the flush – and think that you're upset, angry, shy or confused.

Usually you'll be more aware of the flush than others are. Try checking in a mirror to see if *you* can see it. And try to decide: Is it worse to be thought of as anxious or having a hot flush? We need to have the courage to mention our hot flushes, to break the silence!

Q *Will vitamins or alternative medicines help my hot flushes?*

A Some women do feel that vitamins and supplements provide relief for hot flushes – vitamin E, ginseng root and other remedies are all thought to help although we don't yet have enough information on the best doses to take, and there has been no research as yet to examine the effectiveness of these remedies scientifically.

Remember that some herbal remedies contain small amounts of oestrogen, so if you have been advised not to use oestrogen then you should probably be careful about using these.

Homoeopathy, aromatherapy and acupuncture are all popular holistic approaches to dealing with medical problems generally and often menopausal problems in particular. If you're keen to try any of them to alleviate your hot flushes, make sure you see a registered practitioner (see pages 178 and 179).

If you have a particular problem, then it would be a good idea to get a proper diagnosis first to rule out any serious disease – for instance you should always see your doctor if you have a breast lump or vaginal bleeding after the menopause.

Q *My vagina is drier than usual. Is HRT the only treatment that will help this?*

A First of all, explain to your partner about the effects the menopause can have on vaginal lubrication. HRT can help vaginal dryness but it isn't the only remedy. Often a lubricant such as KY jelly, which is widely available over the counter from chemists, is all you'll need. And there's also a newer product on the market now (called Replens) that can be inserted into the vagina to provide moisture for up to two or three days.

Taking longer over foreplay can also help. And you might want to try making love without penetration for a while, especially if sex has been painful. Pelvic floor exercises increase blood flow to the vagina and help keep it moist (see page 59). Natural live yoghurt applied inside the vagina can be soothing and can help ward off infections, which can cause dryness. If you do want to take HRT specifically for this problem, you can use creams which contain small doses of oestrogen (see page 143), rather than pills or patches.

Remember that there are other things that can cause vaginal dryness – not being sufficiently aroused, for instance, or anxiety or stress, so don't forget to check for these too. Many women experience dryness from time to time for the above reasons before the menopause, so it's as well not to jump to the conclusion that the menopause has caused this problem when you experience it during this time.

Q *I feel low and emotional – is it the menopause or are there any other likely causes?*

A The first step, obviously, is to understand why you feel like this. There are many reasons for feeling distressed and during the menopause it can be hard to make sense of the changes taking place. The commonest causes of feeling low are losing something or someone, not feeling valued, and problems in close relationships at home and at work (see Chapter Two for further information on this).

It might help identify your particular problem if you ask yourself the following questions.

△ When I feel low, what thoughts or problems come to mind?

△ Am I doing too much?

△ Have I recently experienced a loss (it could be a bereavement or a friend moving away)?

△ What in my life gives me self-esteem?

△ Are there any chronic problems or conflicts in my life?

△ What do I, or did I, enjoy?

Sometimes some apparently small change can tip the balance for a busy woman, from coping to feeling overwhelmed. Talk to someone about how you feel. Just putting your concerns into words that another person understands can help. If your family or friends are good listeners, talk to them. If those close to you are part of the problem you may need to see someone else. Ask your doctor for information about counselling

Earning a living can do wonders for your self-esteem and you can do it without even leaving the house – start a needlework course or a cookery class for instance.

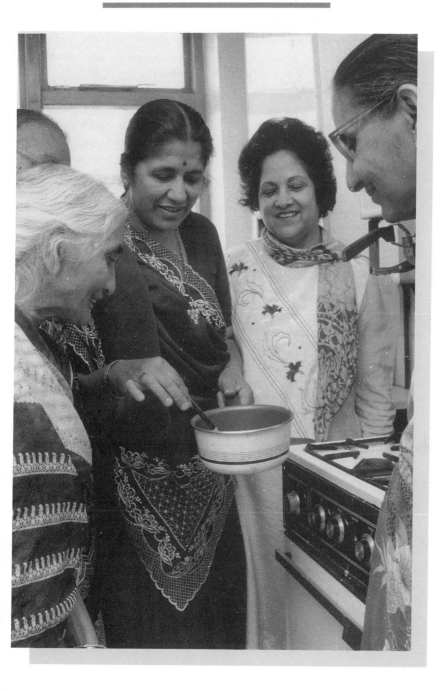

services he or she can recommend; some general practices now have their own counsellor or clinical psychologist available for consultation.

Having lowered oestrogen levels in your body after the menopause does *not* cause depression, but some women do seem to be sensitive to changing or fluctuating hormone levels. There is recent evidence to suggest, however, that stress itself can work to lower hormone levels, which is why, if you're going through the menopause or approaching it, it makes sense to try to reduce stress (see pages 38 to 42).

Don't rush to blame the menopause for problems that might have other causes. Explore other possible reasons, including your reactions to reaching this life-stage. Naturally, to feel sad and sentimental is not abnormal. Use the menopause as a time to make positive changes in your life and try to find ways of dealing with any long-standing problems. If you are very depressed and can't cope, or have no one to talk to, do seek help – we have listed a whole variety of organisations at the end of this book that are there to provide such aid.

Throughout this book we have, explicitly and by implication, stressed the importance of your attitude to yourself.

It is important, for instance, to keep alert to any changes in your body and to stay informed about what is happening to you. Don't be afraid to be assertive – and above all don't hesitate to ask for an explanation of anything that is puzzling or worrying you. If you don't feel it merits a visit to the doctor, contact one of the many organisations that exist in this country to supply support and information for all manner of conditions and situations; you will find a listing of relevant ones at the end of this book.

And a bit of positive thinking can do wonders, too, – not only for the effect it will have on your own morale, looks and health, but also for the effect it can have on the people around you.

This is – to use that old cliche – the first day of the rest of your life so treat it for what it is: a precious gift to enjoy and make the most of. Give yourself the attention you deserve. Keep your health as good as you can, try to eat healthily and take a reasonable amount of exercise; most of all, continue being interested in everything around you.

It's not too late to try something new, so if you think you're getting into a rut – do something about it: learn a language, climb a mountain, go dancing or learn to work a computer. Being involved in things will enable you to meet and talk to people easily and informally, and that can extend your circle of friends and help to keep you stimulated.

Above all, nurture your relationships – with yourself, your family, your partner, your friends: personal happiness can keep you healthy too, particularly during periods of change.

CHAPTER EIGHT

LOOKING BACK AND LOOKING AHEAD

Your path through your menopause will be unique. The specific changes that occur, the way you deal with them, your health and your lifestyle choices, all go to influence your experience of midlife. The menopause is a gateway, and once you are through it you can reach a new equilibrium.

The American anthropologist Margaret Mead coined the term post-menopausal zest to describe the vitality, energy and involvement in life that many women feel after the menopause. Some derive a greater confidence and freedom at this stage of life, and many acquire the ability to free themselves from old stereotypes and gain a whole new sense of self worth.

It helps if you have good health. It helps, too, if you have faced difficulties squarely and attempted to direct the changes in your life. Few changes are easy. But pausing for thought in midlife, looking after yourself, making positive plans and taking a few risks does pay off.

The four women's stories that follow show that there is no one right way, that there is instead a whole series of changes and personal choices.

Good luck!

Carol is a social worker, 55 years old, who had her last period when she was 52.

❝ Looking back, it was harder for me just before the menopause in my mid-40s. My daughter was having problems with her husband and I was very uncertain about my career. I wasn't happy with changes at work. Sam's business was also going through a rocky patch.

I had quite heavy periods. I think I must have been run-down, but I didn't notice it at the time.

I had hot flushes for a few months before I realised that it was the menopause. It took about 18 months for my periods to stop altogether. They seemed to stop and then every few months I'd get another one. Not knowing when it was going to happen was difficult. The flushes continued and I still get one now and again but they were generally not too bad.

For me it was more a case of seeing myself as a menopausal woman. Maybe I thought about that more because my daughter was pregnant at the time. You don't think about wanting to actually have children – it was more about saying good-bye to a very familiar part of me. Again I was pleased not to have heavy periods, although I did feel empty for a while. A bit sad for my womb!

I spoke to one or two people about the menopause because I was curious and I read a lot as well. My family were fine – I think I had more negative ideas about the menopause than they did. That was reassuring. I'm not the type to take tablets. I can see that HRT might be good for some people, but I had no need for it.

I do think that women are freer to be

173

themselves as they get older. You have the courage to be different. I had worked part-time in the same job for over 15 years. It was easy, I suppose, when the children were at home. But two years ago I started to train as a psychotherapist, so I have made a big change of direction.

My health? Well, I eat well and swim twice a week with a friend. I love gardening – that's how I relax. I find it helps me to have varied activities. To divide up my time like this meets my needs and seems to give me energy. 🙶

Veronica is 54, married with three children. Two have left home and one is living at home while studying at a local college. She works as a receptionist in a large firm of accountants.

🙸I had a hysterectomy when I was 47; I'd had a lot of problems with my periods. The doctor left my ovaries when they did the operation. It was odd for me because I wasn't having periods. I think the hormonal menopause came a couple of years later. I had the flushes – which were quite bad for about a year and they made me feel tired; then they tailed off. At that time sex wasn't too good either, because I was tired, I think. But we got through that phase.

The girls in the office did talk about the menopause and their hot flushes. At that time there were a few of us about the same age. We'd laugh and joke and bring fans in to cool down! One or two of them went on HRT and said it helped. How I saw it, was at the time you kept thinking they might stop soon anyway, and for me they did. You do hear of women who get them for years. I suppose I was lucky.

Going through the change hasn't made a big difference to me. I am making an effort with myself though. I've lost a few pounds in weight. It's your attitude that's important, isn't it. My husband and I will both be retiring at about the same time and I'm honestly looking forward to that. I want to do something different. We might move near to the sea – my husband is mad about boats, and I want to get out of the city. 🙶

Molly, 57, lives by herself and runs a small secretarial agency.

🙸I was married for 18 years. The marriage was never very good, we were too similar, both wanting to be in charge. We didn't have any children, mainly because I wasn't confident about the relationship. Eventually we went to marriage guidance. That helped us to talk and to separate amicably.

My life changed most then I suppose, after the divorce. I was 44. Before that I had worked in temporary jobs – a jack of all trades. With John's work we moved around a lot. We sold the house we had and I bought a small flat. I felt terrible for a while but then great relief! I knew I could cope – I've always been quite a strong person.

I started to define my own life, even what I ate. John used to like steaks. I cooked them but now I'm practically a vegetarian. I went into business with a friend. We had a flower shop which did well for a few years.

When my mother died I gave up the shop to stay with my father for a while in Scotland. My sister lived up there as well. I hadn't seen her or her family for a few years.

It was then that my periods started becoming unpredictable and I noticed one or two hot flushes as well. My sister was in her menopause at the same time. It was quite a year for us both. We were very close to our mother and we got a lot out of going through the grief together, as well as the menopause. We went for long walks and talked about life. I'm much closer to her now.

I came back to my flat with renewed enthusiasm and a conviction that my life would be what I made it. After a lot of work I set up my own secretarial agency – which is doing quite well. I take care to dress well. I think that it is important to try to be elegant when you're older. And I'm happy to live alone. I've got used to it. But you need to make the effort to see people and plan weekend breaks. There are a lot more leisure activities catering for my age group now. 🙎

Joyce is 58, married and is a grandmother.

🙎 The change for me lasted for quite a few years. I'm not sure when it started. It happens so gradually, you know. My periods stopped fairly quickly – I was glad about that. I had hot flushes mainly at night. At that time I accepted them.

Although I haven't worked since I had my daughter, I've always been fairly active. I was a school governor and we've always been sociable and done a lot of entertaining. We've got two big dogs and living in the country I get a lot of exercise.

Two things happened to me that led me to see my doctor. Sex had become gradually more painful – I'd read that this could be due to the menopause. Also, and just as important, my mother fractured her hip and was diagnosed as having osteoporosis. As well as organising care for her, I decided that oestrogen was for me! My doctor gave me patches, which are fine. I've had them for two years now although I had to try a couple of different tablets (progestogens) before we found one to suit me. But I feel good now. At least I feel as if I'm doing

175

something to protect my bones. The bleeding with the tablets is fairly light and for me it's worth it.

In general, I do feel quite a bit wiser with age. I don't feel the need to please other people all the time like I used to. I think I get more respect as a result, too. Stan and I get on, we know each other so well. At this stage you can accept each others strengths and weaknesses.

My priorities and interests are rather different now, too. I've become more active in a local environmental group; I enjoy my grandchild very much; and I've also taken up the piano again — picked up where I left off at 15! 99

USEFUL ORGANISATIONS

If you wish to receive information from any of the organisations listed below, please send a stamped addressed envelope with your enquiry.

ASH (Action on Smoking and Health)
109 Gloucester Place, London WIN 3PH
Telephone 071 935 3519
8 Frederick Street, Edinburgh EH2 2HB
Telephone 031 225 4725
372A Cowbridge Road, Canton, Cardiff CF5 IHF
Telephone 022 641101
Ulster Cancer Foundation, 40 Eglantine Avenue, Belfast BT9 6DX
Telephone 0232 663281

ALCOHOLICS ANONYMOUS
PO Box I, Stonebow House, Stonebow, York YOI 2NJ
Telephone 0904 644026
Baltic Chambers, 50 Wellington Street, Glasgow G2 6HJ
Telephone 041 221 9027
The Central Office, 152 Lisburn Road, Belfast BT9 6AJ
Telephone 0232 681084

AL-ANON
Family Groups, 61 Great Dover Street, London SEI 4YP
Telephone 071 403 0888
Baltic Chambers, 50 Wellington Street, Glasgow G2 6HJ
Telephone 041 221 7356
Room 8, Cathedral Buildings, 64 Donegal Street, Belfast
Telephone 0232 243489

THE AMARANT TRUST

80 Lambeth Road, London SE1 7PW
Telephone 071 401 3855
Provides information about HRT and advice on midlife issues.

ARTHRITIS CARE

18 Stephenson Way, London NW1 2HD
Telephone 071 916 1500

BEREAVEMENT

For counselling contact your local community health council or health
centre or your local MIND group. If you live in London, contact The
London Bereavement Projects Coordinating Group, c/o 68 Chalton
Street, London NW1 1JR
Telephone 071 388 2153

BIRMINGHAM WOMEN'S COUNSELLING AND THERAPY CENTRE

The Uffculne Clinic, Queensbridge Road, Moseley,
Birmingham B13 8QD
Telephone 021 455 8677

BREAST CARE AND MASTECTOMY ASSOCIATION

15–19 Britten Street, London SW3 3TZ
Telephone 071 867 1103

THE BRITISH ACUPUNCTURE ASSOCIATION AND REGISTER

179 Gloucester Place, London NW1 6DX
Telephone 071 724 5330

BRITISH ASSOCIATION FOR COUNSELLING

37A Sheep Street, Rugby, Warwickshire CV21 3BX
Telephone 50788 78328

BRITISH ASSOCIATION OF PSYCHOTHERAPISTS
37 Mapesbury Road, London NW2 4HJ
Telephone 081 452 9823

BRITISH DIABETIC ASSOCIATION
10 Queen Anne Street, London W1M OBD
Telephone 071 323 1531

BRITISH HOMOEOPATHIC ASSOCIATION
27a Devonshire Street, London W1N 1RJ
Telephone 071 935 2163

BRITISH NATUROPATHIC AND OSTEOPATHIC ASSOCIATION
6 Netherhall Gardens, London NW3 5RR
Telephone 071 435 8728

BRITISH SPORTS ASSOCIATION FOR THE DISABLED
Solecast House, 13–27 Brunswick Place, London N1 6DX
Telephone 071 490 4919

BROOK ADVISORY CENTRE
233 Tottenham Court Road, London W1P PAE
Telephone 071 580 2991
2 Lower Gilmore Place, Edinburgh EH3 9NY
Telephone 031 229 3596
Offers family planning contraception advice for women of all ages.

CARE (CANCER AFTER-CARE & REHABILITATION SOCIETY)
21 Zetland Road, Redland, Bristol BS6 7AH
Telephone 0272 427419

CAREER COUNSELLING SERVICES
46 Ferry Road, London SW13 9PW
Telephone 081 741 0335

CAREERS FOR WOMEN
2 Valentine Place, London SE1 8QH
Telephone 071 401 2280
Offers career counselling for women.

CARERS NATIONAL ASSOCIATION
29 Chilworth Mews, London W2 3RG
Telephone 071 724 7776

CHEST, HEART AND STROKE ASSOCIATION
142 Grassmarket, Edinburgh EH1 2GU
Telephone 031 225 5002
21 Dublin Road, Belfast BT2 7FG
Telephone 0232 320184
For England see Stroke Association later in this listing.

CORONARY PREVENTION GROUP
102 Gloucester Place, London W1H 3DA
Telephone 071 935 2889

CRUSE-BEREAVEMENT CARE
126 Sheen Road, Richmond, Surrey TW9 1UR
Telephone 081 940 4818
3 Rutland Square, Edinburgh EH1 2AS
Telephone 031 229 6275
1st Floor, 50 University Street, Belfast BT7 1FY
Telephone 0232 232695

DIABETES FOUNDATION
177A Tennison Road, London SE25 5NF
Telephone 081 656 5467

EATING DISORDERS ASSOCIATION
Sackville Place, 44/48 Magdalen Street, Norwich NR3 1JE
Telephone 0603 621414

ENDOMETRIOSIS SOCIETY
245a Coldharbour Lane, London SW9 8RR
Telephone 071 737 0380

ETHNIC MINORITIES ADVICE BUREAU
1a Station Road, London SE25 5AH
Telephone 081 653 6505

FAMILY PLANNING ASSOCIATION
27–35 Mortimer Street, London WIN 7RJ
Telephone 071 636 7866
4 Museum Place, Cardiff CFI 3BG
Telephone 022 142766
113 University Street, Belfast BT7 1HP
Telephone 0232 325488

HEALTH EDUCATION AUTHORITY
Hamilton House, Mabledon Place, London WC1H 9TX
Telephone 071 383 3833
Offers details of local community health councils throughout the country.

THE HEALTH EDUCATION BOARD FOR SCOTLAND
Woodburn House, Canaan Lane, Edinburgh EH10 4SG
Telephone 031 447 8044

HERPES ASSOCIATION
41 North Road, London N7 9DP
Telephone 071 609 9061

HYSTERECTOMY SUPPORT NETWORK
c/o 3 Lynne Close, Green Street Green, Orpington, Kent

LESBIAN AND GAY SWITCHBOARD
Telephone 071 837 7324
Offers 24–hour information and advice service for gay women.

181

MENOPAUSE

There are menopause clinics throughout the UK. Check with your local Well-Woman Clinic, Family Planning Clinic or the gynaecology department of your local hospital for one near you. If there isn't one in your area, check with The Amarant Trust (see address and telephone number on page 178) for information on any private facilities in your area or town.

MIND (NATIONAL ASSOCIATION FOR MENTAL HEALTH)

22 Harley Street, London W1N 2ED
Telephone 071 637 0741
MIND provides information and answers queries about counselling or psychiatric services.

NATIONAL ASSOCIATION FOR THE CHILDLESS

St George's Rectory, Tower Street, Birmingham B19 3UY
Telephone 021 359 4887

NATIONAL ASSOCIATION OF WIDOWS

54/57 Allison Street, Digbeth, Birmingham B5 5TH
Telephone 021 643 8348

NATIONAL COUNCIL FOR ONE-PARENT FAMILIES

255 Kentish Town Road, London NW5 2RX
Telephone 071 267 1361
Offers confidential advice about social services, housing and maintenance.

NATIONAL FEDERATION OF SELF-HELP ORGANISATIONS

150 Townmead Road, London SW6 2RA
Telephone 071 731 8440

NATIONAL OSTEOPOROSIS SOCIETY

PO Box 10, Radstock, Bath, Avon BA3 3YB
Telephone 0761 432472

PRE-RETIREMENT ASSOCIATION OF GREAT BRITAIN AND NORTHERN IRELAND

The Nodus Centre, University Campus, Guildford, Surrey GU2 5RX
Telephone 0483 39323
Coordinates county and regional groups throughout the United Kingdom. Contact above for the addresses and telephone numbers of your local group.

RELATE: NATIONAL MARRIAGE GUIDANCE

Herbert Gray College, Little Church Street, Rugby,
Warwicks. CV21 3AP
Telephone 0788 573241

SAMARITANS

10 The Grove, Slough, Berks. SL1 1QP
Telephone 0753 532713

SCOTTISH MARRIAGE GUIDANCE COUNCIL

26 Frederick Street, Edinburgh EH2 2JR
Telephone 031 825 5006

SCOTTISH RETIREMENT COUNCIL

204 Bath Street, Glasgow G2 4HL
Telephone 041 332 9427

ASSOCIATION TO AID THE PERSONAL AND SEXUAL RELATIONSHIPS OF PEOPLE WITH A DISABILITY (SPOD)

286 Camden Road, London N7 0BJ
Telephone 071 607 8851

183

STROKE ASSOCIATION
CHSA House, Whitecross Street, London EC1Y 8GJ
Telephone 071 490 7999

VEGAN SOCIETY
7 Battle Road, St. Leonards-on-Sea, East Sussex TN37 7AA
Telephone 0424 427393

VEGETARIAN SOCIETY OF THE UK LTD
Parkdale, Dunham Road, Altrincham, Cheshire WA14 4QG
Telephone 061 928 0793

WOMEN'S COUNSELLING AND THERAPY SERVICE
15 Harold Road, Shirley, Southampton
Telephone 0703 337530

WOMEN'S HEALTH AND REPRODUCTIVE RIGHTS CENTRE
52 Featherstone Street, London EC1Y 8RT
Telephone 071 251 6580/6332

WOMEN'S NATIONAL CANCER CONTROL CAMPAIGN
Suna House, 128 Curtain Road, London EC2A 3AR
Telephone 071 729 1735

WOMEN'S THERAPY CENTRE
6–9 Manor Gardens, London N7 6LA
Telephone 071 263 6200
Runs individual therapy sessions and also groups dealing with eating problems.

YOGA FOR HEALTH FOUNDATION
Ickwell Bury, near Biggleswade, Bedfordshire SG18 9ES
Telephone 0767 627271

BIBLIOGRAPHY

FOR MENOPAUSE, MIDLIFE, AGEING

The Menopause: Coping with the Change Jean Coope (Optima, 1984)
Your Menopause: Prepare Now for a Positive Future Myra Hunter (Pandora, 1990)
Menopause Naturally Sadja Greenwood (Volcano Press, 1984)
HRT: Your Questions Answered Val Godfree and Malcolm Whitehead (Penguin, 1992)
The Change Germaine Greer (Penguin, 1992)
Change of Life: A Psychological Study of Dreams and the Menopause Ann Mankowitz (Inner City Books, 1984)
Prime Time Helen Franks (Pan, 1981)
Growing Older, Living Longer Teresa Hunt (The Bodley Head, 1988)
 – a critical look at attempts at rejuvenation.
Ourselves Growing Older J Shapiro (Fontana, 1989)
The Silent Passage Gail Sheehy (Random House, 1991)

SEX, RELATIONSHIPS AND EMOTIONAL PROBLEMS

Women's Experience of Sex Sheila Kitzinger (Penguin, 1985)
The Relate Guide to Sex and Loving Relationships Sarah Litvinoff (Vermilion, 1992)
Safer Sex, the Guide for Women Today Diane Richardson (Pandora, 1990)
Overcoming your Nerves Tony Lake (Sheldon Press, 1982)
Fears, Phobias and Panic Maureen Sheehan (David Fulton, 1988)
Coping with Stress: A Woman's Guide Dr Georgia Witkin-Lancil (Sheldon Press, 1985)
You and Your Adolescent Laurence Steinberg and Ann Levine (Vermilion, 1992)
Living with a Drinker: How to Change Things Mary Wilson (Pandora, 1989)

In Our Own Hands Sheila Ernst and Lucy Goodison (The Women's Press, 1981 – a book of self-help therapy).

Dealing with Depression Kathy Nairne and Gerrilyn Smith (The Women's Press, 1984)

Depression: The Way Out of Your Prison Dorothy Rowe (Routledge, 1983)

A Woman in Your Own Right Anne Dickson (Quartet Books, 1982) – about how to be assertive.

You Just Don't Understand Deborah Tannen (Virago, 1992)

FOR LIFESTYLES, LIFE CHANGES

Guide to Healthy Eating Health Education Authority leaflet (free)

Living with Stress Cary Cooper, Rachel Cooper and Lynn Eaker (Penguin, 1988) – deals with work and other stresses

Stress and Relaxation Jane Madders (Optima, 1979)

Relax: Dealing with Stress Murray Watts and Cary Cooper (BBC Books, 1992)

So You Want to Stop Smoking Health Education Authority leaflet (free)

Stopping Smoking Made Easier Martin Raw (Health Education Authority leaflet, 1992)

Women under the Influence Brigid McConville (Grafton, 1991) – about women alcoholics

Exercise: Why Bother Sports Council/Health Education Authority (free)

Yogacise Lyn Marshall (BBC Books, 1993)

Eva Fraser's Facial Workout (Penguin, 1991)

What Every Woman Should Know about her Breasts Dr Patricia Gilbert (Sheldon Press, 1986)

Contraception: The Facts Peter Bromwich and Tony Parsons (Oxford Medical Publications, 1984)

What To Do When Someone Dies Which Consumer Guides (Hodder & Stoughton, 1991)

Bereavement Colin Murray Parkes (Pelican, 1975)

186

COPING WITH COMMON PROBLEMS

Everywoman: A Gynaecological Guide for Life Derek Llewellyn (Penguin, revised edition 1992)

The Well-Woman Dr Margery Morgan (BBC Books, 1992)

Why Suffer? Periods and their Problems Lynda Byrne and Katy Gardner (Virago, 1982)

The Experience of Infertility Naomi Pfeffer and Anne Woollett (Virago, 1983)

Positive Smear Susan Quillam (Penguin, 1989)

Endometriosis Suzie Hayman (Penguin, 1991)

In Control: Coping With Incontinence Penny Mares (Age Concern, 1990)

Thrush Caroline Clayton (Sheldon Press, 1984)

The New Our Bodies Ourselves Boston Women's Health Collective (Penguin, 1989)

Natural Healing for Women Susan Curtis and Romy Fraser (Pandora, 1991)

An Alternative Health Guide Brian Inglis and Ruth West (Michael Joseph, 1983)

Get a Better Night's Sleep Ian Oswald and Kirstine Adam (Optima, 1983)

Experiences of Hysterectomy Ann Webb (Optima, 1989)

Thyroid Disorders Dr Rowan Hillson (Optima, 1991)

Coping with Rheumatoid Arthritis Robert Philips (Avery, 1988)

Coping with Osteoarthritis Robert Philips (Avery, 1989)

INDEX

188